THIRD EDITION

Bates' Pocket Guide to
PHYSICAL EXAMINATION
AND HISTORY TAKING

Lynn S. Bickley, MD
Associate Professor of Medicine and Neuropsychiatry
Departments of Internal Medicine and Neuropsychiatry
Health Sciences Center
Texas Tech University
Lubbock, Texas

Robert A. Hoekelman, MD
Professor Emeritus of Pediatrics
University of Rochester School of Medicine and Dentistry
Rochester, New York

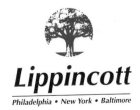

Lippincott
Philadelphia • New York • Baltimore

Acquisitions Editor: Ilze Rader
Editorial Assistant: Dale Thuesen
Managing Editor: Barbara Ryalls
Senior Production Manager: Helen Ewan

Production Coordinator: Mike Carcel
Design Coordinator: Doug Smock
Indexer: Katherine Pitcoff

Library of Congress Cataloging-in-Publication Data

Bickley, Lynn S.
    Bates' pocket guide to physical examination and history taking / Lynn S. Bickley, Robert A. Hoekelman. — 3rd ed.
        p.   cm.
    Rev. ed. of: A pocket guide to physical examination and history taking / Barbara Bates, Lynn S. Bickley, Robert A. Hoekelman. 2nd ed. ©1995.
    Includes bibliographical references and index.
    ISBN 0–7817–1869–4 (alk. paper)
    1. Physical diagnosis Handbooks, manuals, etc. 2. Medical history taking Handbooks, manuals, etc. I. Hoekelman, Robert A. II. Bates, Barbara, 1928–   Pocket guide to physical examination and history taking. III. Title. IV. Title: Pocket guide to physical examination and history taking.
    [DNLM: 1. Medical History Taking Handbooks. 2. Physical Examination—methods Handbooks. WB 39 B583b 2000]
RC76.B38   2000
616.07'54—dc21
DNLM/DLC
for Library of Congress   99–38243
                                                     CIP

Care has been taken to confirm the accuracy of the information presented and to describe generally accepted practices. However, the authors, editors, and publisher are not responsible for errors or omissions or for any consequences from application of the information in this book and make no warranty, express or implied, with respect to the contents of the publication.

The authors, editors and publisher have exerted every effort to ensure that drug selection and dosage set forth in this text are in accordance with current recommendations and practice at the time of publication. However, in view of ongoing research, changes in government regulations, and the constant flow of information relating to drug therapy and drug reactions, the reader is urged to check the package insert for each drug for any change in indications and dosage and for added warnings and precautions. This is particularly important when the recommended agent is a new or infrequently employed drug.

Some drugs and medical devices presented in this publication have Food and Drug Administration (FDA) clearance for limited use in restricted research settings. It is the responsibility of the health care provider to ascertain the FDA status of each drug or device planned for use in their clinical practice.

DEDICATION

To Barbara Bates,

whose clarity of thought and dialogue with readers and colleagues have illuminated the techniques of physical examination and interviewing and guided students to mastery for more than two decades

CONTENTS

The Musculoskeletal System

The Nervous System

Clinical Data

CHAPTER 6

CLINICAL THINKING AND THE PATIENT'S RECORD   *247*

INTRODUCTION

The *Pocket Guide to Physical Examination and History Taking,*
3E is a concise, portable text that

- Outlines the health history
- Provides an illustrated review of the physical
  examination
- Reminds students of some common findings
- Describes some of the special techniques of assessment
  that the student may need in specific instances but may
  not recall in sufficient detail
- Provides succinct aids to interpretation of selected
  findings

This edition marks a publication milestone as the *Pocket
Guide* passes from Barbara Bates, MD, to a new editor and
author, Lynn Bickley, MD. Dr. Bates has created a landmark
text in the field of physical diagnosis and interviewing, with
standards of accuracy and clarity recognized by students
worldwide. We honor her achievement and continue her
tradition of excellence.

There are several ways to use the *Pocket Guide:*

- To review and thus remember the content of a health
  history.
- To review and rehearse the techniques of examination.
  This can be done while learning a single section and
  again while combining the approaches to several body
  systems or regions into an integrated examination.
- To review some common variations of normal and
  some selected abnormalities. Observation is more
  astute when the examiner knows what to look, listen,
  and feel for.
- To look up special techniques as the need arises.
  Maneuvers such as everting an eyelid or doing an

Allen test are included in the relevant sections of the examination and are initiated by a shaded red bar. This bar helps readers to use or ignore the special techniques, as they prefer.
• To look up additional information about possible findings, including abnormalities and standards of normal.

The *Pocket Guide* is not intended to serve as a primary text from which to learn the skills of taking a history or performing a physical examination. Its detail is insufficient for these purposes. It is intended instead as a mechanism for review and recall and as a convenient, brief, and portable reference.

In the third edition, we have added new material in musculoskeletal examination to assist in assessing sports-related injuries and changes of aging. New photographs clarify changes of diabetic retinopathy and hallmarks of malignant melanoma. We have also introduced new tables in Chapter 2 to enhance Health Promotion and Counseling. Other tables have been expanded or reused. The purposes and recommended uses of the book remain the same.

THE HEALTH HISTORY

Taking a history is usually the first and often the most important part of your interaction with patients. You gather much of the data on which diagnoses are based, you learn about the patients as people and how they experience their symptoms and illnesses, and you begin to establish a trusting relationship.

There are several ways to facilitate these objectives. Try to provide an environment that is private, quiet, and free of interruption. Seat yourself in a location that is agreeable to the patient, and make sure that he or she is comfortable. Address the patient by name and title, e.g., Mrs. Green, and introduce yourself.

Start the history with open-ended questions: "What brings you to the hospital? . . . Anything else? . . . Tell me about it." Additional ways of encouraging patients to tell their stories include:

Facilitation—posture, actions, or words that communicate
    interest, such as leaning forward, making eye contact,
    or saying "Mm-hmmm" or "Go on"
Reflection—repetition of a word or phrase that a patient
    has used
Clarification—asking what the patient meant by a word or
    phrase
Empathic responses—recognizing through actions or words
    the feelings of a patient, such as offering a tissue or
    saying "I understand" or "That must have been
    frightening"

Asking about feelings that a patient has had regarding
    symptoms, events, or other matters

Interpretation—putting into words what you infer about
    the patient's feelings or about the meaning to the
    patient of symptoms, events, or other matters

To get specific details, direct questions are often necessary.

- Word them in language understandable to the patient.
- Express them neutrally so as not to bias the patient.
- Ask about one item at a time.
- Proceed from the general to the specific.
- Ask for graded responses rather than a simple yes or
  no. Multiple-choice questions may also be used.

Some topics may initially be difficult for clinicians to ask
about or for patients to discuss, but are very important to include in any history. These include violence and abuse, depression and thoughts of suicide, the use of alcohol and
drugs, sexual practices, and sexually transmitted diseases.
Review and practice approaches to these topics to be able to
explore them effectively.

A COMPREHENSIVE HISTORY OF AN ADULT

DATE AND TIME of the history

IDENTIFYING DATA: age, gender, ethnicity, place of birth,
marital status, occupation, and religion

SOURCE OF REFERRAL, if any

SOURCE of the history

RELIABILITY of the history

CHIEF COMPLAINT(S)

PRESENT ILLNESS: a clear, chronological narrative that in-
cludes the onset of the problem, the setting in which it developed, its manifestations, and any treatments. The princi-
pal symptoms should be described in terms of their seven
basic attributes:

- Location
- Quality
- Quantity or severity
- Timing (onset, duration, frequency)
- Setting
- Factors that aggravate or relieve
- Associated manifestations

Note negative data that may have diagnostic significance.

The present illness should also include the patient's understanding of symptoms and incapacities, his or her responses to them, and the meaning and impact that they hold for the patient's life.

Medications, including home remedies, nonprescription drugs, vitamin/mineral supplements, and borrowed medicines, with doses and frequency of use

Allergies, including specific reaction

PAST HISTORY

Childhood Illnesses

Adult Illnesses, including medical, surgical, obstetric/gynecologic, and psychiatric illnesses

Accidents and Injuries

Transfusions

CURRENT HEALTH STATUS

Tobacco, with type, amount, and duration of use

Alcohol, Drugs, and Related Substances

Exercise and Diet, including frequency of exercise and usual daily intake of food and beverages

Immunizations, such as tetanus, pertussis, diphtheria, polio, measles, rubella, mumps, influenza, hepatitis B, *Hemophilus influenzae,* type B, and pneumococcal vaccine

Screening Tests, such as tuberculin test, Pap smears, mammograms, cholesterol levels, stools for occult blood

Safety Measures (such as seat belts)

Environmental Hazards, at home, school, and workplace

FAMILY HISTORY

- Age and health, or age and cause of death, of parents, siblings, spouse, and children. Data on other relatives may also be useful.
- The occurrence of diabetes, heart disease, hypercholesterolemia, high blood pressure, stroke, kidney disease, tuberculosis, cancer, arthritis, anemia, allergies, asthma, headaches, epilepsy, mental illness, alcoholism, drug addiction, and symptoms like those of the patient

PERSONAL AND SOCIAL HISTORY

Occupation and Education

Home Situation and Significant Others, including family and friends

Daily Life over a 24-hour period

Important Experiences, including upbringing, school, military service, work, financial situation, marriage, retirement

Leisure Activities and Hobbies

Religious Affiliations and Beliefs relevant to perceptions of health, illness, and treatment

REVIEW OF SYSTEMS

General. Usual weight, recent weight change, fatigue, fever, sleep patterns or insomnia

Skin. Rashes, lumps, sores, itching, dryness, color change, changes in hair or nails

Head. Headaches, head injury

Eyes. Vision, glasses, or contact lenses, last eye examination, pain, redness, excessive tearing, double vision, spots, specks, flashing lights, glaucoma, cataracts

Ears. Hearing acuity, tinnitus, vertigo, earaches, infection, discharge

Nose and Sinuses. Frequent colds; nasal stuffiness, discharge, itching; hay fever, nosebleeds, sinus trouble

Mouth and Throat. Condition of teeth and gums, bleeding gums, last dental examination, sore tongue, frequent sore throats, hoarseness

Neck. Lumps in the neck, "swollen glands," goiter, pain or stiffness in the neck

Breasts. Lumps, pain or discomfort, nipple discharge, self-examination

Respiratory. Cough, sputum (color, quantity), hemoptysis, wheezing, asthma, bronchitis, emphysema, pneumonia, tuberculosis, pleurisy; last chest x-ray

Cardiac. Heart failure, high blood pressure, rheumatic fever, heart murmurs; chest pain or discomfort, palpitations; dyspnea, orthopnea, paroxysmal nocturnal dyspnea, edema; past ECG or other heart tests

Gastrointestinal. Trouble swallowing, heartburn, appetite, nausea, vomiting, regurgitation, vomiting of blood, indigestion. Frequency of bowel movements, color and size of stools, change in bowel habits, rectal bleeding or black tarry stools, hemorrhoids, constipation, diarrhea. Abdominal pain, food intolerance, excessive belching or passing of gas. Jaundice, liver or gallbladder trouble, hepatitis

Urinary. Frequency of urination, polyuria, nocturia, burning or pain on urination, hematuria, urgency, reduced caliber or force of the urinary stream, hesitancy, incontinence; urinary infections, stones

Genital, Male

- Hernias, penile discharge or sores, testicular pain or masses, any sexually transmitted diseases and their

treatments, exposure to HIV infection, precautions taken against it and other STDs
- Sexual interest, orientation, function, satisfaction, and problems; contraceptive methods

Genital, Female
- Age at menarche; regularity, frequency, and duration of periods; amount of bleeding, bleeding between periods or after intercourse, last menstrual period; dysmenorrhea; premenstrual tension; age at menopause, menopausal symptoms, postmenopausal bleeding
- Discharge, itching, sores, lumps, any sexually transmitted diseases and their treatments, exposure to HIV infection, precautions taken against it and other STDs
- Number of pregnancies, number and type of deliveries, number of abortions (spontaneous and induced); complications of pregnancy; contraceptive methods
- Sexual interest, orientation, function, satisfaction; any problems, including dyspareunia

Peripheral Vascular. Intermittent claudication, leg cramps, varicose veins, clots in the veins, Raynaud's disease (phenomenon)

Musculoskeletal. Muscle or joint pains, stiffness, arthritis, gout, backache. If present, describe the location and associated symptoms (swelling, redness, pain, tenderness, stiffness, weakness, limitation of motion or activity).

Neurologic. Fainting, blackouts, seizures, weakness, paralysis, numbness, tingling, tremors or other involuntary movements, attention span

Hematologic. Anemia, easy bruising or bleeding, past transfusions and possible reactions

Endocrine. Thyroid trouble, heat or cold intolerance, excessive sweating; diabetes, excessive thirst or hunger, polyuria

Psychiatric. Nervousness, tension, mood including depression; any suicidal ideation; memory

A COMPREHENSIVE PEDIATRIC HISTORY

The child's history follows the same outline as the adult's history, with certain *additions* presented here.

IDENTIFYING DATA: Date and place of birth; nickname; first names of parents (and last name of each, if different)

CHIEF COMPLAINTS. Determine if they are the concerns of the child, the parent(s), a schoolteacher, or some other person.

PRESENT ILLNESS. Determine how each member of the family responds to the child's symptoms, why he or she is concerned, and the secondary gain the child may get from the illness.

PAST HISTORY

Birth History, important when neurologic or developmental problems are present. Get hospital records if necessary.

- Prenatal—maternal health: medications, tobacco, drug, and alcohol use, vaginal bleeding, weight gain, duration of pregnancy
- Natal—nature of labor and delivery, birth weight, Apgar scores at 1 and 5 minutes
- Neonatal—resuscitation efforts, cyanosis, jaundice, infections; nature of bonding

Feeding History, important with under- and overnutrition

- Breast feeding—frequency and duration of feeds, difficulties encountered; timing and method of weaning
- Artificial feeding—type; amount, frequency; vomiting, colic, diarrhea; vitamins, iron, and fluoride supplements; introduction of solid foods
- Eating habits—likes and dislikes, types and amounts of food eaten; parental attitudes and response to feeding problems

Growth and Development History, important with delayed

growth, psychomotor and intellectual retardation, and behavioral disturbances

- Physical growth—weight, height, and head circumference at birth and 1, 2, 5, and 10 years; periods of slow or rapid growth
- Developmental milestones—ages child held head up, rolled over, sat, stood, walked, and talked
- Social development—day and night sleeping patterns; toilet training; speech problems; habitual behaviors, discipline problems; school performance; relationships with parents, siblings, and peers

CURRENT HEALTH STATUS

Allergies. Pay particular attention to childhood allergies—eczema, urticaria, perennial allergic rhinitis, asthma, food intolerance, and insect hypersensitivity.

Immunizations. Include dates given and any untoward reactions.

Screening Tests. Include those for vision, hearing, cholesterol, tuberculosis, blood lead, sickle cell disease, and inborn errors of metabolism.

2

HEALTH PROMOTION AND COUNSELING

MENTAL STATUS

DEPRESSION
- Screen for low self-esteem, anhedonia, sleep disorder, difficulty concentrating or making decisions—especially if patient is young, female, single, divorced, seriously or chronically ill, or bereaved

SUICIDE
- Screen for suicidal ideation, intent, especially if patient is adolescent or young, or with history of psychiatric illness, substance abuse, personality disorder, prior suicide attempt, family history of suicide

DEMENTIA
- Screen for memory deficits, loss of orientation to place, impoverished speech or word-finding difficulty, change in behavior or daily functioning, especially if positive family history
- Assess effects of medications, possible depression, metabolic abnormalities
- Educate and counsel family members

SKIN

- Counsel to avoid unnecessary sun exposure, use sunscreen with SPF-15
- Teach "ABCDE" screen for dysplastic

nevi/melanomas: **A**symmetry,
irregular **B**orders, variation in **C**olor,
Diameter >6 mm, **E**levation

- Survey skin: 3-year intervals ages
20–39, annually >40

HEAD AND NECK

VISUAL ACUITY
- Assess visual acuity (J-point card,
Snellen chart)

- Adults >65, screen for cataracts
(clouding of lens), macular
degeneration (mottling of macula,
variation in retinal pigmentation,
subretinal hemorrhage or
exudate), glaucoma (increased cup-to-
disc ratio)

HEARING
- Ask about hearing loss, especially if
>65 or if history of congenital or
familial deafness, syphilis, rubella,
meningitis, exposure to hazardous
noise levels at work

- Test hearing by audioscope, tuning
fork >"whisper" test, rubbing fingers

ORAL HEALTH
- Inspect oral cavity for tooth decay,
gingivitis, periodontal disease; check
also for ulcerations, leukoplakia

- Review medications for risk of
decreased salivary flow

- Recommend annual dental visits,
fluoride toothpaste/flossing,
avoidance of tobacco and refined
sugars

THORAX AND LUNGS

SMOKING
CESSATION
- Promote smoking cessation
using the "4A's":
Ask about smoking

Advise stopping in clear personalized
message
Assist setting stop date
Arrange and monitor follow-up,
counseling, possible nicotine
replacement

CARDIOVASCULAR SYSTEM

CHOLESTEROL
- Check cholesterol age 20, every 5 years (men ages 35–65, women ages 45–65); lipid profile when cholesterol >220–240 or other risk factors

DIET, EXERCISE, WEIGHT
- Promote diet modification, regular exercise, body weight <20% upper limit of normal (see tables pp. 139–140)

BLOOD PRESSURE
- Promote optimal blood pressure control (see page 191)

BREASTS AND AXILLAS

BREAST CANCER
- Teach monthly self-breast exam
- Exam breasts yearly after age 40 or as indicated by prior or family history
- Recommend mammogram: annually ages 50–65; baseline age 40 or if family history age 35; at 1–2 year intervals ages 40–50 (controversial)

ABDOMEN

HEPATITIS
- Screen for alcoholism, risk of infectious hepatitis, risk of colon cancer

- Recommend vaccination for hepatitis when indicated:

    Hepatitis A—travelers, food handlers, military and health care personnel, child-care workers

    Hepatitis B—young adults not

previously immunized, injection drug users and their sexual partners, patients with sexually transmitted diseases or frequent transfusions, travelers to endemic areas

- Screen for colorectal cancer (recommendations controversial), especially if family history of polyps, colorectal cancer, adenoma, or if personal history of ulcerative colitis, polyps, or endometrial, ovarian or breast cancer. If >50, consider annual fecal occult blood test (FOBT), screening sigmoidoscopy every 3–5 years, possibly alternating with barium enema

MALE AND FEMALE GENITALIA

HIV, STD
INFECTION

- Screen carefully for infection with HIV, sexually transmitted diseases (STDs)
- Educate about transmission of HIV, STDs, and protective practices
- Test for HIV if increased risk, injection drug use, history of blood transfusions before 1985

PLANNING OF
PREGNANCY

- Educate about timing of ovulation and relationship to pregnancy

CERVICAL CANCER

- Perform Pap smear: annually after age 18 or if sexually active; more frequently if HIV, human papillomavirus, history of STDs. If Pap smears negative, annually × 3 years, test at 3-year intervals until 65 (controversial); test after 65 if recent abnormal Pap smear, risk factors, or incomplete screening

MENOPAUSE

- Assess and counsel about menopause and hormone replacement therapy

PREGNANCY

NUTRITION; EXERCISE	• Promote adequate nutrition, appropriate exercise
DOMESTIC VIOLENCE	• Assess attitudes about pregnancy, screen for domestic violence

ANUS, RECTUM, PROSTATE

PROSTATE CANCER	• Review prostate cancer risk factors. If over 50, discuss pros and cons of digital rectal exam (DRE) and testing with prostate specific antigen (PSA)
	• If warranted, DRE and PSA annually after 50, or after 40 if African American or positive family history (guidelines controversial)
COLORECTAL CANCER	• See "Abdomen" regarding FOBT and screening sigmoidoscopy
	• Consider DRE annually after age 50 (guidelines controversial)

PERIPHERAL VASCULAR SYSTEM

PERIPHERAL VASCULAR DISEASE	• Recommend health-promoting lifestyle (exercise, diet, blood pressure control, smoking cessation)
	• Assess symptoms if claudication; palpate peripheral pulses, inspect legs and feet for pale color, absence of hair

MUSCULOSKELETAL SYSTEM

OSTEOPOROSIS	• Recommend health-promoting lifestyle, especially exercise to strengthen skeleton (see above)

- Review need for calcium and vitamin D supplements
- Assess need for biphosphonates, hormone replacement therapy (women)
- Consider bone densitometry

FALLS
- Assess gait, posture; deficits in cognition, vision, proprioception; risk of osteoporosis, medications affecting balance or cognition

NERVOUS SYSTEM

STROKE
- Control blood pressure
- Recommend risk-factor reduction for atherosclerosis—smoking cessation, diabetes control, cholesterol reduction if needed
- Assess and treat transient ischemic attacks

This table presents general guidelines for health promotion and counseling. Controversy regarding selected guidelines is indicated. Readers are encouraged to pursue further discussions in additional sources such as the U.S. Preventive Health Services Task Force Guide to Clinical Preventive Services *(1996) and* Health Promotion and Disease Prevention in Clinical Practice, *eds. S.H. Woolf, S. Jonas, & R.S. Lawrence (1996).*

3

THE PHYSICAL EXAMINATION OF AN ADULT

OVERVIEW

For a comprehensive physical examination, use a sequence that maximizes your efficiency and minimizes the patient's effort, yet allows you to be thorough. One such sequence is outlined below, together with symbols that indicate the patient's positions.

Key to the Symbols for the Patient's Position

○— Lying supine

○⌐ Lying on left side (left lateral decubitus)

○⌐ Lying on right side

○— Lying supine, with head of bed raised to 30°

○⌐ Same, turned partly to left side

⋀⋀ Lying supine, with hips flexed, abducted, and externally rotated, and knees flexed (lithotomy position)

♀ Sitting

♀ Sitting, leaning forward

♀ Standing

♀ Squatting

Each symbol pertains until a new one appears. Two symbols separated by a slash indicate either or both positions.

For the first three sections of this examination, no specific position is necessary.

SEQUENCE OF A COMPREHENSIVE EXAMINATION

General Survey

Mental Status

Skin

Head and Neck, including an initial survey of respiration; can include cranial nerves

Posterior Thorax and Lungs

Musculoskeletal Examination of the neck and upper back; costovertebral angle tenderness

Breast Inspection, Axillae, and Epitrochlear Nodes

Musculoskeletal Examination of the temporomandibular joint and upper extremities, if indicated

Anterior Thorax and Lungs

Breast Palpation

Cardiovascular System

- For finding an elusive apical impulse and for hearing a left-sided S_3 or S_4 and the murmur of mitral stenosis

- For hearing the murmur of aortic regurgitation

Abdomen

Legs and Feet: peripheral vascular and musculoskeletal examination, and inspection for neurologic findings (position, muscle bulk, involuntary movements)

∘⫫⊱ Neurologic System in detail if indicated:

- Cranial nerves not yet examined

- Motor system: muscle bulk, muscle tone, strength, rapid alternating movements, point-to-point movements

- Sensory system

- Reflexes

⌇ Varicose Veins

Spine, Legs, and Feet

Male: Genitalia and Hernias

Gait, Romberg test, pronator drift

∘⊥ Male: Rectum

∿∿ Female: Genitalia and Rectum

The rest of this chapter is devoted to the examination, unit by unit. To facilitate the review or rehearsal of individual body systems or regions, each is described as a whole. The Thorax and Lungs, for example, make up one unit. In practice, however, as shown in the overview above, examination of the breasts and axillae is interposed between the examinations of the posterior thorax and the anterior thorax. Such interpositions or other changes in sequence are indicated by colored shading in the following text.

Special techniques that may not be used often are placed at the end of units and are set off by a gray bar. You may find them there or skip them according to your purpose.

Examination Techniques   Possible Findings

THE GENERAL SURVEY

Check vital signs at outset or later in examination. **Observe** the rest of the following attributes during the interview or examination.

Apparent State of Health	Robust, acutely or chronically ill, frail
Signs of Distress	Labored breathing, wincing, sweatiness, trembling
Skin Color	Pallor, cyanosis, jaundice
Height and Build	Tall, short, muscular; disproportionately long limbs
Sexual Development	Facial hair, voice changes, breast development
Weight, by appearance or measurement	Emaciated, slender, plump, fat
Posture, Motor Activity, and Gait	Postures to ease breathing or pain; ataxia, a limp, paralysis
Dress, Grooming, and Personal Hygiene	Excessive clothes of hypothyroidism, long sleeves to cover a rash or needle marks
Odors of Body or Breath	Alcohol, odors of diabetic acidosis, uremia, liver failure
Facial Expression	Stare of hyperthyroidism, immobile face of parkinsonism

Examination Techniques	Possible Findings
Speech	Fast speech of hyperthyroidism, hoarseness of myxedema
Vital Signs, including	
• Pulse rate and blood pressure	Tachycardia, hypertension
• Respiratory rate	Tachypnea
• Temperature	Fever, hypothermia

MENTAL STATUS

Observe patient's mental status throughout your interaction. **Test** specific functions if indicated during the interview or physical examination.

APPEARANCE AND BEHAVIOR

Assess the following:

Level of Consciousness. **Observe** patient's alertness and response to verbal and tactile stimuli.	Normal consciousness, lethargy, obtundation, stupor, coma
Posture and Motor Behavior. **Observe** pace, range, character, and appropriateness of movements.	Restlessness, agitation, bizarre postures, immobility, involuntary movements
Dress, Grooming, and Personal Hygiene	Fastidiousness, neglect

Examination Techniques	Possible Findings
Facial Expressions during rest and interaction	Anxiety, depression, elation, anger, responses to imaginary people or objects, withdrawal
Manners, Affect, and Relation to Persons and Things	

SPEECH AND LANGUAGE

Note quantity, rate, loudness, clarity, and fluency of speech. If indicated, test for aphasia.	Aphasia, dysphonia, dysarthria, changes with mood disorders

MOOD

Ask about patient's spirits. **Note** nature, intensity, duration, and stability of any abnormal mood. If indicated, **assess** risk of suicide.	Happiness, elation, depression, anxiety, anger, indifference

THOUGHT AND PERCEPTIONS

Thought Processes. **Assess** logic, relevance, organization, and coherence of patient's thought.	Derailments, flight of ideas, incoherence, confabulation, blocking
Thought Content. **Ask** about and explore any unusual or unpleasant thoughts.	Obsessions, compulsions, delusions, feelings of unreality
Perceptions. **Ask** about any unusual perceptions, e.g., seeing or hearing things.	Illusions, hallucinations
Insight and Judgment. **Assess** patient's insight into the illness and the level of judgment used in making decisions or plans.	Recognition or denial of the mental cause of symptoms; bizarre, impulsive, or unrealistic judgment

Examination Techniques   Possible Findings

COGNITIVE FUNCTIONS

If indicated, **assess:**

Orientation to time, place, and person

Disorientation

Attention

- *Digit span*—the ability to repeat a series of numbers forward and then backward

- *Serial 7s*—the ability to subtract 7 repeatedly, starting with 100

- *Spelling backward* of a five-letter word, such as W-O-R-L-D

Poor performance of digit span, serial 7s, and spelling backward is common in dementia and delirium but has other causes too.

Remote Memory, e.g., birthdays, anniversaries, social security number, schools, jobs, wars

Impaired in late stages of dementia

Recent Memory, e.g., events of the day

Recent memory and new learning ability impaired in dementia, delirium, and amnestic disorders

New Learning Ability—the ability to repeat three or four words after a few minutes of unrelated activity

Examination Techniques	Possible Findings

HIGHER COGNITIVE FUNCTIONS

If indicated, **assess:**

Information and Vocabulary. **Note** range and depth of patient's information, complexity of ideas expressed, and vocabulary used. For the fund of information you may also ask names of presidents, other political figures, or large cities.

These attributes reflect intelligence, education, and cultural background. They are limited by mental retardation, but fairly well preserved in early dementia.

Calculating Abilities, such as addition, subtraction, and multiplication

Poor calculation in mental retardation and dementia

Abstract Thinking—the ability to respond abstractly to questions about
- The meaning of *proverbs,* such as "A stitch in time saves nine"
- The *similarities* of beings or things, such as a cat and a mouse or a piano and a violin

Concrete responses (observable details rather than concepts) common in mental retardation, dementia, and delirium. Responses sometimes bizarre in schizophrenia

Constructional Ability. **Ask** patient

Impaired ability common in dementia and with parietal lobe damage

- To copy figures such as circle, cross, diamond, and box, and two intersecting pentagons, or

- To draw a clock face with numbers and hands

Examination Techniques	Possible Findings

THE SKIN

Examine each region.

SKIN

Inspect and **palpate. Note**

- Color — Cyanosis, jaundice, carotenemia, changes in melanin

- Moisture — Moist, dry, oily

- Temperature — Cool, warm

- Texture — Smooth, rough

- Mobility—the ease with which a fold of skin can be moved — Decreased in edema

- Turgor—the speed with which the fold returns into place — Decreased in dehydration

Note any lesions and their

- Anatomic location — Generalized, localized

- Arrangement — Linear, clustered, dermatomal

- Type — Macule, papule, pustule, bulla, tumor

- Color — Red, white, brown, mauve

NAILS

Inspect and **palpate** the fingernails and toenails.

Examination Techniques	**Possible Findings**

Note

- Color
- Shape
- Any lesions

Cyanosis, pallor

Clubbing

Paronychia, onycholysis

HAIR

Inspect and **palpate** the hair. **Note**

- Quantity
- Distribution
- Texture

Thin, thick

Patchy or total alopecia

Fine, coarse

THE HEAD AND EYES

HEAD

Examine the

- Hair, including quantity, distribution, and texture

Coarse and sparse in myxedema, fine in hyperthyroidism

- Scalp, including lumps or lesions

Pilar cysts, psoriasis

- Skull, including size and contour

Hydrocephalus, skull depression from trauma

- Face, including symmetry and facial expression

Facial paralysis, emotions

- Skin, including color, texture, hair distribution, and lesions

Pale, fine, hirsute

Acne, skin cancer

Examination Techniques	Possible Findings

EYES

Test visual acuity in each eye.

Diminished acuity

Assess visual fields, if indicated.

Hemianopsia, quadrantic defects

Inspect the

- Position and alignment of eyes

  Exophthalmos, strabismus

- Eyebrows

  Seborrheic dermatitis

- Eyelids

  Sty, chalazion, ectropion, ptosis, xanthelasma

- Lacrimal apparatus

  Swollen lacrimal sac

- Conjunctiva and sclera

  Red eye, jaundice

- Cornea, iris, and lens

  Corneal opacity, cataract

Examine pupils for

- Size, shape, and symmetry

  Miosis, mydriasis, anisocoria

- Reactions to light, and, if these are abnormal—

  Absent in 3rd nerve paralysis

- The near reaction

  Useful in tonic pupils, Argyll Robertson pupils

Assess the extraocular muscles by observing

- The corneal reflections from a midline light

  Muscular imbalance

Examination Techniques	Possible Findings
• The six cardinal directions of gaze	Paralytic or nonparalytic strabismus, nystagmus, lid lag

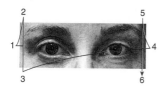

• Convergence	Poor in hyperthyroidism

Inspect the fundi with an ophthalmoscope, including the

• Red reflex	Cataracts, artificial eye
• Optic disc	Papilledema, glaucomatous cupping, optic atrophy

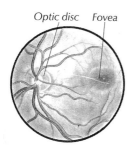

Optic disc   Fovea

• Arteries, veins, and A–V crossings	Hypertensive changes
• Adjacent retina. **Note** any lesions.	Hemorrhages, exudates, cotton-wool patches, microaneurysms, pigmentation

Examination Techniques	Possible Findings
• Macular area	Macular degeneration
• Anterior structures	Vitreous floaters, cataracts

THE EARS

Examine, on each side:

THE AURICLE
Inspect it.   Keloid, epidermoid cyst

If you suspect otitis,

• Move the auricle up and down, and press on the tragus.	Causes pain in otitis externa
• Press firmly behind the ear.	May be tender in otitis media and mastoiditis

THE EAR CANAL AND EARDRUM
Pull the auricle up, back, and slightly out.

Inspect, through an otoscope speculum,

• The canal	Cerumen, otitis externa
• The eardrum, as illustrated on the next page 34.	Acute otitis media, serous otitis media, tympano-sclerosis, perforations

Examination Techniques   **Possible Findings**

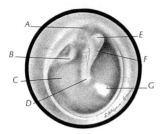

A = *Pars flaccida*   B = *Incus*
C= *pars tensa*   D = *Umbo*
E= *Short process of malleus*
F= *Handle of malleus*
G = *Cone of light*

(After Hawke M, Keene M, Alberti PW: Clinical Otoscopy: A Text and
Colour Atlas. Edinburgh, Churchill Livingstone, 1984)

HEARING

Assess auditory acuity to
whispered or spoken voice.

If hearing is diminished,
use a 512-Hz tuning fork to

These tests help to
distinguish between
sensorineural and
conduction hearing loss.

- Test lateralization
  (**Weber test**)

- Compare air and bone
  conduction (**Rinne test**)

NOSE AND SINUSES

Inspect the external nose.

Inspect, through a
speculum, the

Examination Techniques	Possible Findings
• Nasal mucosa that covers the septum and turbinates, noting its color and any swelling	Swollen and red in viral rhinitis, swollen and pale in allergic rhinitis; polyps; ulcer from cocaine use
• Nasal septum for position and integrity	Deviation, perforation
Palpate the sinuses for tenderness:	Tender in acute sinusitis
• Frontal	
• Maxillary	

MOUTH AND PHARYNX

Inspect the

• Lips	Cyanosis, pallor, cheilosis
• Oral mucosa	Canker sores
• Gums	Gingivitis, periodontal disease
• Teeth	Dental caries, tooth loss
• Roof of the mouth	Torus palatinus
• Tongue, including	
Papillae	Glossitis
Symmetry	12th cranial nerve paralysis
Any lesions	Cancer of tongue
• Floor of the mouth	Cancer

Examination Techniques	**Possible Findings**

- Pharynx, including

  Color or any exudate — Pharyngitis

  Presence and size of tonsils — Tonsillitis, peritonsillar abscess

  Symmetry of the soft palate as patient says "ah" — 10th cranial nerve paralysis

NECK

Inspect the neck. — Scars, masses, torticollis

Palpate the lymph nodes. — Cervical lymphadenopathy due to inflammation, malignancy

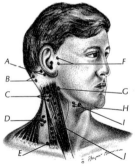

A = Posterior auricular
B = Occipital   C = Superficial cervical   D = Posterior cervical
E = Supraclavicular
F = Preauricular   G = Tonsillar
H = Submental
I = Submandibular   J = Deep cervical chain

Inspect and **palpate** the position of the trachea. — Deviated trachea

Examination Techniques	Possible Findings

Inspect the thyroid gland.   Goiter, nodules

- At rest

- As patient swallows
  water

From behind patient, **palp-**   Goiter, nodules, tenderness
ate the thyroid gland, in-   of thyroiditis
cluding the isthmus and the
lateral lobes, as illustrated
below.

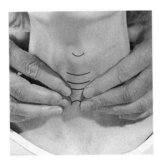

FEELING THE ISTHMUS

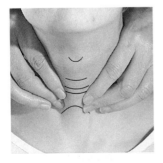

FEELING THE LATERAL LOBES

Examination Techniques	Possible Findings

- At rest

- As patient swallows water

The initial survey of respiration may be done while examining the front of the neck. After feeling the thyroid gland from behind, you may proceed to a musculoskeletal examination of the neck and upper back and a check for costovertebral angle tenderness.

SPECIAL TECHNIQUES

EVERSION OF THE UPPER EYELID. The patient should relax and look down.

Eversion of lid reveals foreign bodies and lesions of the palpebral conjunctiva of upper lid.

Grasp eyelashes of upper lid and pull them gently down and forward.

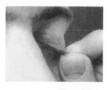

Place an applicator stick or the edge of a tongue blade horizontally on upper lid at least 1 cm above lid margin, and push it down on eyelid, thus everting lid.

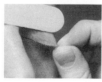

Hold lashes of upper lid against eyebrow while you inspect the palpebral conjunctiva.

When finished, pull eyelashes gently forward, and ask patient to look up.

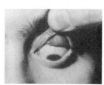

Examination Techniques	Possible Findings

ʅ   FOR NASOLACRIMAL DUCT OBSTRUCTION. As patient looks up, press on lower lid near medial canthus and just inside rim of bony orbit. Look for fluid coming out of puncta into eye.

Regurgitation of mucopurulent fluid from puncta suggests obstructed duct and may identify cause of excessive tearing. Avoid this test if area is inflamed and tender.

THE THORAX AND LUNGS

ʅ   SURVEY

Inspect the thorax and its respiratory movements. **Note**

- Rate, rhythm, depth, and effort of breathing

  Tachypnea, hyperpnea, Cheyne–Stokes breathing

- Inspiratory retraction of the supraclaviclar areas

  Occurs in COPD, asthma, upper airway obstruction

- Inspiratory contraction of the sternomastoids

  Indicates severe breathing difficulty

Observe shape of patient's chest.

Normal or barrel chest

Listen to patient's breathing for

- Stridor

  Stridor in upper airway obstruction from foreign body or epiglottitis

- Wheezes

  Wheezes in obstructive lung disease

THE POSTERIOR CHEST

Inspect the chest for

Examination Techniques	Possible Findings
• Deformities or asymmetry	Kyphoscoliosis
• Abnormal inspiratory retraction of the interspaces	Retraction in airway obstruction
• Impairment or unilateral lag in respiratory movement	Disease of the underlying lung or pleura, phrenic nerve palsy

Palpate the chest for

• Tender areas	Fractured ribs
• Assessment of visible abnormalities	Masses, sinus tracts
• Respiratory expansion	Impairment, one or both sides
• Tactile fremitus	Local or generalized decrease or increase

Percuss the chest in the areas illustrated, comparing one side with the other at each level.	Dullness occurs when fluid or solid tissue replaces normally air-filled lung. Hyperresonance often accompanies emphysema or pneumothorax.

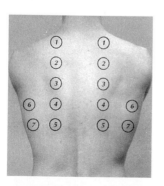

Examination Techniques	Possible Findings
Identify level of diaphragmatic dullness on each side and **estimate** diaphragmatic excursion.	Pleural effusion or a paralyzed diaphragm raises level of dullness.

Listen to chest with stethoscope in areas shown above, again comparing sides.

- Evaluate the breath sounds.

  Vesicular, bronchovesicular, or bronchial breath sounds; decreased breath sounds from decreased air flow

- Note any adventitious (added) sounds.

  Crackles (fine and coarse) and continuous sounds (wheezes and rhonchi)

Observe their qualities, place in the respiratory cycle, and location on the chest wall. Do they clear with deep breathing or coughing?

Assess transmitted voice sounds if you have heard bronchial breath sounds in abnormal places. Ask patient to

- Say "99" and "ee"

  Bronchophony, egophony, and whispered pectoriloquy

- Whisper "99" or "1, 2, 3"

While the patient is still sitting, you may inspect the breasts and examine the axillary and epitrochlear lymph nodes. Also examine the temporomandibular joint and the musculoskeletal system of the upper extremities.

Examination Techniques   **Possible Findings**

o— THE ANTERIOR CHEST

Inspect the chest for

- Deformities or asymmetry   Pectus excavatum

- Intercostal retraction   From obstructed airways

- Impaired or lagging   Disease of the underlying
  respiratory movement   lung or pleura, phrenic
                           nerve palsy

Palpate the chest for

- Tender areas   Tender pectoral muscles,
                 costochondritis

- Assessment of visible   Flail chest
  abnormalities

- Respiratory expansion

- Tactile fremitus

Percuss the chest in the   Normal cardiac dullness
areas illustrated   may disappear in emphy-
                               sema.

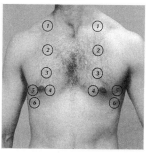

Listen to chest with
stethoscope. **Note**

- Breath sounds

Examination Techniques	Possible Findings

- Adventitious sounds

- If indicated, transmitted voice sounds

SPECIAL TECHNIQUES

ASSESSMENT OF PULMONARY FUNCTION. If appropriate, walk with patient down the hall or up a flight of stairs. Observe rate, effort, and sound of breathing, and inquire about symptoms.

FORCED EXPIRATORY TIME. Ask patient to take a deep breath in and then breathe out as quickly and completely as possible, with mouth open. Listen over trachea with diaphragm of stethoscope and time audible expiration. Try to get three consistent readings, allowing rests as needed.

If the patient understands and cooperates well, a forced expiratory time of 6 or more seconds strongly suggests obstructive pulmonary disease.

IDENTIFICATION OF A FRACTURED RIB. Point tenderness of a rib suggests fracture but may be due to soft-tissue injury. With one hand on patient's sternum and the other on the thoracic spine, squeeze patient's chest. Does this anteroposterior compression cause pain? If so, where?

An increase in local rib pain, distant from your hands, suggests rib fracture rather than just soft-tissue injury.

Examination Techniques   **Possible Findings**

THE BREASTS AND AXILLAE

⅋ FEMALE BREASTS

Inspect the breasts for

• Size and symmetry	Development, asymmetry
• Contour	Flattening, dimpling
• Appearance of the skin	Edema (peau d'orange) in breast cancer

Inspect the nipples.

• Compare their size, shape, and direction of pointing	Inversion, retraction, deviation
• Note any rashes, ulcer-ations, or discharge.	Paget's disease of the nipple, galactorrhea

Continue your inspection as patient

• Raises both arms above her head	Dimpling and abnormalities of contour
• Presses her hands against her hips	

○— **Palpate** the breasts for

• Consistency	Physiologic nodularity
• Tenderness	Infection, premenstrual tenderness
• Nodules. If present, **note** their	Cyst, fibroadenoma, cancer

Examination Techniques   Possible Findings

Location

Size

Shape

Consistency

Delimitation

Tenderness

Mobility

Palpate each nipple.   Thickening in cancer

♀/♂ **MALE BREASTS**

Inspect the nipple and   Gynecomastia, cancer
areola.

Palpate the areola and   Gynecomastia, cancer, fat
adjacent area.

♀   **AXILLAE**

Inspect for rashes, infection,   Hidradenitis suppurativa,
and pigmentation.   acanthosis nigricans

Palpate the central   Lymphadenopathy
axillary nodes.

If indicated, **palpate** the
other axillary nodes:

• Pectoral group

• Lateral group

• Subscapular group

Examination Techniques	Possible Findings

S P E C I A L   T E C H N I Q U E

○— BREAST DISCHARGE.
Compress the areola in a
spokelike pattern around
the nipple if patient has
reported spontaneous
nipple discharge. **Watch**
for discharge.

Type and source of
discharge may thereby be
identified.

THE CARDIOVASCULAR SYSTEM

○— THE ARTERIAL PULSE
RADIAL ARTERY

Palpate the radial pulse.
Note

- Heart rate

  Tachycardia, bradycardia

- Rhythm. If this is
  irregular, listen to
  the heart.

  Premature contractions,
  atrial fibrillation

CAROTID ARTERY

Palpate the carotid artery
pulse. **Note**

- Amplitude

  Increased, decreased

- Any variations in
  amplitude

  Pulsus alternans

- Contour

  Bounding upstroke and
  rapid fall in aortic
  regurgitation

Listen with a stethoscope
for a bruit or a murmur
transmitted from the heart.

Bruit and possible thrill in
carotid obstruction;
transmitted murmur of
aortic stenosis

Examination Techniques	Possible Findings

BLOOD PRESSURE

Estimate systolic blood pressure by palpation and **add** 30 mm Hg. Use this sum as the target for further cuff inflations.

This step helps you to detect an auscultatory gap.

Measure blood pressure with a sphygmomanometer.

If indicated, **check** it

Orthostatic (postural) hypotension

JUGULAR VEINS

Identify the jugular venous pulsations and their highest point in the neck. Adjust angle of bed as necessary.

Measure jugular venous pressure—the vertical distance between this highest point and the sternal angle, normally less than 3–4 cm.

Elevated venous pressure in right-sided heart failure

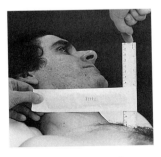

Study the venous pulse waves.

Absent *a* waves in atrial fibrillation; prominent *v* waves in tricuspid regurgitation.

Examination Techniques   **Possible Findings**

THE HEART

Inspect and **palpate** the anterior chest for pulsations.

Identify the apical impulse. Turn patient to left as necessary. **Note**

- Location of impulse

  Displaced to left in pregnancy.

- Diameter

  Increased diameter, amplitude, and duration in left ventricular enlargement

- Amplitude

- Duration

Feel for a right ventricular impulse in left parasternal and epigastric areas.

Prominent impulses suggest right ventricular enlargement.

Palpate left and right second interspaces close to sternum. **Note** any thrills in these areas.

Pulsations of great vessels; accentuated S_2; thrills of aortic or pulmonic stenosis

Listen to heart with stethoscope. Use its diaphragm in all areas illustrated on page 49 and its bell at the apex and the lower left sternal border.

Examination Techniques   Possible Findings

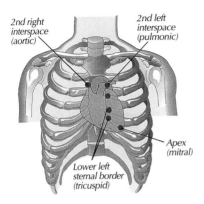

2nd right interspace (aortic)

2nd left interspace (pulmonic)

Apex (mitral)

Lower left sternal border (tricuspid)

Listen at each area for:

- S_1

- S_2. Is splitting normal in left 2nd and 3rd interspaces?

  Physiologic (inspiratory) or pathologic (expiratory) splitting

- Extra sounds in systole

  Systolic clicks

- Extra sounds in diastole

  S_3, S_4

- Systolic murmurs

  Midsystolic, pansystolic, late systolic murmurs

- Diastolic murmurs

  Early, mid-, or late diastolic murmurs

Identify, if murmurs are present, their

- Timing in the cardiac cycle (systole, diastole)

Examination Techniques	Possible Findings
• Shape	Plateau, crescendo, decrescendo
• Location of maximal intensity	
• Radiation	
• Intensity on a 6-point scale	
• Pitch	High, medium, low
• Quality	Blowing, harsh, musical, rumbling

Listen at the apex with patient turned toward left side.

Left-sided S_3, S_4, and diastolic murmur of mitral stenosis

Listen down left sternal border to the apex as patient sits, leaning forward, with breath held in exhalation.

Diastolic decrescendo murmur of aortic regurgitation

S P E C I A L   T E C H N I Q U E S

PULSUS ALTERNANS. Feel pulse for alternation in amplitude. Lower pressure of blood pressure cuff slowly to systolic level while you listen with stethoscope over brachial artery.

Alternating amplitude of pulse or sudden doubling of Korotkoff sounds indicates a pulsus alternans—a sign of left ventricular failure.

PARADOXICAL PULSE. Lower pressure of blood pressure cuff slowly and note two pressure levels:

A difference greater than 10 mm Hg signifies a paradoxical pulse. Consider obstructive lung disease, pericardial

Examination Techniques	**Possible Findings**
(1) where Korotkoff sounds are first heard, and (2) where they first persist through the respiratory cycle. These levels are normally not more than 3–4 mm Hg apart.	tamponade, or constrictive pericarditis.
ᴑ VALSALVA MANEUVER. Ask patient to strain down. In suspected *mitral valve prolapse (MVP)*, listen to the timing of click and murmur.	Ventricular filling decreases, and the systolic click of MVP becomes earlier, and the murmur lengthens.
To distinguish *aortic stenosis (AS)* from *hypertrophic cardiomyopathy (HC)*, listen to the intensity of the murmur.	In AS, the murmur decreases; in HC, it often increases.
⚥/⚲ SQUATTING AND STANDING. In suspected *MVP*, listen for the click and murmur in both positions.	Squatting increases ventricular filling, and delays the click and murmur. Standing reverses the changes.
Try to distinguish *AS* from *HC* by listening to the murmur in both positions.	Squatting increases murmur of AS and decreases murmur of HC. Standing reverses the changes.

THE ABDOMEN

ᴑ— **Inspect** the abdomen, including	
• Skin	Scars, striae, veins
• Umbilicus	Hernia, inflammation

Examination Techniques	**Possible Findings**
• Contours for shape, symmetry, enlarged organs or masses	Bulging flanks, suprapubic bulge, large liver or spleen, tumors
• Any peristaltic waves	GI obstruction
• Any pulsations	Increased in aortic aneurysm
Auscultate the abdomen, if indicated clinically, for	
• Bowel sounds	Increased or decreased motility
• Bruits	Bruit of renal artery stenosis

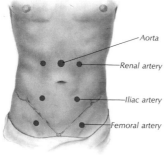

Aorta
Renal artery
Iliac artery
Femoral artery

• Friction rubs	Liver tumor, splenic infarct
Percuss the abdomen for patterns of tympany and dullness	Ascites, GI obstruction, pregnant uterus, ovarian tumor
Palpate all quadrants of the abdomen	
• Lightly for guarding, rebound, and tenderness	Peritoneal inflammation

Examination Techniques	Possible Findings

- Deeply for masses or tenderness

Tumors, a distended viscus

THE LIVER

Percuss span of liver dullness in midclavicular line (MCL).

Hepatomegaly

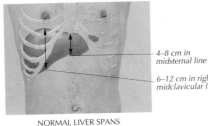

4–8 cm in midsternal line

6–12 cm in right midclavicular line

NORMAL LIVER SPANS

Feel the liver edge, if possible, as patient breathes in.

Firm edge of cirrhosis

Measure its distance from the costal margin in the MCL.

Increased in hepatomegaly

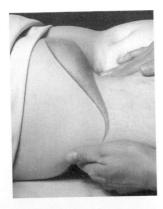

Examination Techniques	Possible Findings

Note any tenderness or masses.

Tender liver of hepatitis or congestive heart failure; tumor mass

THE SPLEEN

Percuss across left lower anterior chest, noting change from tympany to dullness.

Check for a splenic percussion sign.

Try to **feel** spleen with the patient:

Splenomegaly

• Supine

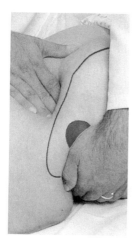

⊶   • Lying on the right side

Examination Techniques   **Possible Findings**

○— THE KIDNEYS

Try to **palpate** each kidney.   Enlargement from cysts, cancer, hydronephrosis

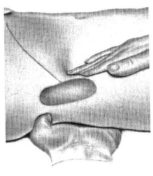

⌐ **Check** for costoverte-   Tender in kidney infection
bral angle tenderness.

○— THE AORTA

Palpate the aorta's pulsations and, in older people,
estimate its width.

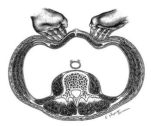   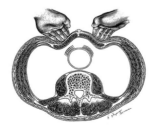

ABDOMINAL AORTA   **AORTIC ANEURYSM**

Examination Techniques   **Possible Findings**

S P E C I A L   T E C H N I Q U E S

⊶ REBOUND TENDER-
NESS. Press slowly on a tender area, then quickly with-
draw your hand. Greater
pain on withdrawal is re-
bound tenderness.

Rebound tenderness
suggests peritoneal
inflammation

⊶/⊶ SHIFTING DULL-
NESS IN ASCITES. Map areas
of tympany and dullness
with patient supine and
lying on side. (see below)

Ascitic fluid usually shifts
to dependent side,
changing the margin of
dullness. (see below)

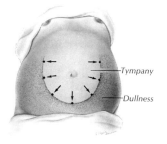

Tympany

Dullness

Tympany

Dullness

⊶ FLUID WAVE IN AS-
CITES. Ask patient or an assistant to press edges of
both hands into midline of
abdomen. Tap one side,
and feel for a wave transmitted to the other side.

A palpable wave suggests
but does not prove ascites.

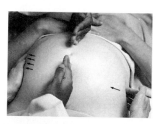

Examination Techniques   **Possible Findings**

o— HOOKING TECH-
NIQUE FOR PALPATING
LIVER. Stand to right of patient's chest and place both
hands side by side with fingers below lower border of
liver dullness. Press in and
up and try to feel liver as patient breathes in.

A liver that is not palpable
by the usual method is
sometimes felt this way.

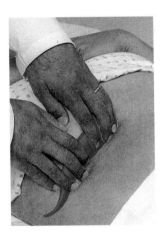

o— MURPHY'S SIGN FOR
ACUTE CHOLECYSTITIS.
Hook your thumb under
right costal margin at edge
of rectus muscle, and ask
patient to take a deep
breath.

Sharp tenderness and a
sudden stop in inspiratory
effort constitutes a positive
sign.

Examination Techniques	**Possible Findings**

o— BALLOTTEMENT. To find an organ or mass in an ascitic abdomen, try to ballotte it. Place your stiffened and straightened fingers on the abdomen, briefly jab them toward the structure, and try to touch its surface.

Your hand, quickly displacing the fluid, stops abruptly as it touches the solid surface.

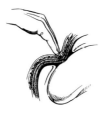

o— ASSESSING POSSIBLE APPENDICITIS, the basic approach:

In classic appendicitis:

"Where did the pain begin?"   Near the umbilicus

"Where is it now?"   Right lower quadrant

Ask patient to cough.
"Where does it hurt?"   Right lower quadrant

Search for local tenderness.   RLQ tenderness

Feel for muscular rigidity.   RLQ rigidity

Perform a rectal exam and, in women, a pelvic exam.   Possibly local tenderness, especially if appendix is retrocecal

Examination Techniques   **Possible Findings**

MALE GENITALIA

This examination is usually deferred until the patient is standing

Wear gloves

☂ THE PENIS

Inspect the

• Development of the penis and the skin and hair at its base	Sexual maturation, lice
• Prepuce	Phimosis
• Glans	Balanitis, chancre, herpes, warts, cancer
• Urethral meatus	Hypospadias, discharge of urethritis

Palpate

• Any visible lesions	Chancre, cancer
• The shaft	Urethral stricture or cancer

THE SCROTUM AND ITS CONTENTS

Inspect

• Contours of scrotum	Hernia, hydrocele, cryptorchidism
• Skin of scrotum	Rashes

Examination Techniques	Possible Findings

Palpate each

- Testis, noting any

  Lumps   Cancer

  Tenderness   Orchitis, torsion

- Epididymis   Epididymitis, cyst

- Spermatic cord and   Varicocele
  adjacent areas

HERNIAS

Inspect inguinal and
femoral areas as patient
strains down.

Inguinal and femoral
hernias

Palpate external inguinal
ring through scrotal skin,
and ask patient to strain
down.

Indirect and direct inguinal
hernias

S P E C I A L   T E C H N I Q U E

TRANSILLUMINA-
TION OF A SCROTAL
MASS. Darken room, and
shine beam of a good flashlight from behind scrotum
through mass. Note whether
mass lights up with a red
glow.

Fluid-filled masses such as
cysts light up; those
containing blood or solid
tissue do not.

Examination Techniques	**Possible Findings**

ANUS, RECTUM, AND PROSTATE—MALE

Inspect the

- Sacrococcygeal area

  Pilonidal cyst or sinus

- Perianal area

  Hemorrhoids, warts, herpes, chancre, cancer

Palpate the anal canal and rectum with a lubricated and gloved finger. Feel the

- Walls of the rectum

  Cancer of the rectum, polyps

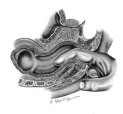

- Prostate gland, as shown below

  Benign hyperplasia, cancer, acute prostatitis

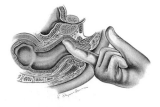

Try to **feel** above the prostate for irregularities or tenderness, if indicated.

Rectal shelf of peritoneal metastases; tenderness of inflammation

Examination Techniques   Possible Findings

FEMALE GENITALIA, ANUS, AND RECTUM

Wear gloves.

EXTERNAL GENITALIA

o— **Observe** pubic hair to   Normal or delayed puberty
assess sexual maturity.

∿∿ **Inspect** the external
genitalia.

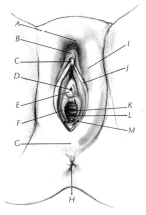

*A = Mons pubis   B = Prepuce
C= Clitoris   D = Urethral orifice
E= Opening of Skene's gland
F= Vestibule   G = Perineum
H= Anus   I = Labium majus
J= Labium minus   K = Hymen
L= Vagina   M = Opening of
Bartholin's gland*

- Labia   Inflammation

- Clitoris   Enlarged in masculinization

- Urethral orifice   Urethral caruncle

- Introitus   Imperforate hymen

Examination Techniques	Possible Findings
Palpate for enlargement or tenderness of Bartholin's glands.	Bartholin's gland infection
Milk the urethra for discharge, if indicated.	Discharge of urethritis

INTERNAL EXAMINATION

Locate the cervix with a gloved and water-lubricated index finger.

Assess support of vaginal outlet by asking patient to strain down.

Cystocele, cystourethrocele, rectocele

Enlarge the introitus by pressing its posterior margin downward.

Insert a water-lubricated speculum of suitable size, starting with speculum held obliquely.

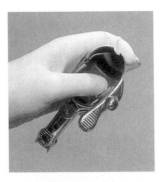

ENTRY ANGLE

Examination Techniques   Possible Findings

Rotate speculum, open it
and inspect cervix.

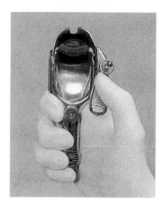

ANGLE AT FULL INSERTION

Observe

- Position

  Cervix faces forward if
  uterus is retroverted.

- Color

  Purplish in pregnancy

- Epithelial surface

  Squamous and columnar
  epithelium

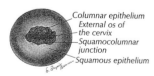

- Any discharge or
  bleeding

  Discharge from os in
  mucopurulent cervicitis

- Any ulcers, nodules, or
  masses

  Herpes, polyp, cancer

Examination Techniques	Possible Findings
Obtain specimens for cytology (Pap smears) with	Early cancer before it is clinically evident
• An endocervical swab and a spatula to scrape the ectocervix	
• Or, if the woman is not pregnant, a cervical brush for a combined specimen	
Inspect the vaginal mucosa as you withdraw the speculum.	Bluish color and deep rugae in pregnancy; vaginal cancer
Palpate the cervix and fornices.	Pain on moving cervix in pelvic inflammatory disease
Palpate, by means of a bimanual examination,	
• The uterus	Pregnancy, myomas; soft isthmus in early pregnancy
• Right and left adnexa	Ovarian masses, salpingitis, tubal pregnancy
Assess strength of pelvic muscles. With your vaginal fingers clear of the cervix, ask patient to tighten her muscles around your fingers as hard and long as she can.	A firm squeeze that compresses your fingers, moves them up and inward, and lasts more than 3 seconds is full strength.
Perform a rectovaginal examination.	Retroverted uterus

Examination Techniques	Possible Findings

oʒ/ʌʌ ANUS AND RECTUM

Inspect the anus.   Hemorrhoids

Palpate the anal canal and   Rectal cancer, normal uter-
rectum.   ine cervix or tampon (felt
                                        through the rectal wall)

S P E C I A L   T E C H N I Q U E

HERNIAS. Ask the pa-
tient to strain down, as you
palpate for a bulge in

• The femoral canal   Femoral hernia

• The labia majora up to   Indirect inguinal hernia
  just lateral to the pubic
  tubercle

THE PERIPHERAL VASCULAR SYSTEM

Inspection of the limbs may also include findings relevant to the musculoskeletal and nervous systems.

⌐ ARMS

Inspect for

• Size and symmetry, any   Lymphedema, venous
  swelling   obstruction

• Venous pattern   Venous obstruction

• Color and texture of   Raynaud's disease
  skin and nails

Examination Techniques	**Possible Findings**

Palpate the pulses:

- Radial   Lost in thromboangiitis obliterans or acute arterial occlusion

- Brachial

Feel for the epitrochlear nodes.   Lymphadenopathy from local cuts, infections

o— **LEGS**

Inspect for

- Size and symmetry, any swelling   Venous insufficiency, lymphedema

- Venous pattern   Varicose veins

- Color and texture of skin   Pallor, rubor, cyanosis

- Hair distribution   Loss in arterial insufficiency

Check for pitting edema.   Peripheral or systemic causes of edema

Palpate the pulses: Loss of pulses in acute arterial occlusion and arteriosclerosis obliterans

- Femoral
- Popliteal
- Dorsalis pedis
- Posterior tibial

Palpate the inguinal lymph nodes: Lymphadenopathy

Examination Techniques   **Possible Findings**

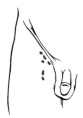

- Horizontal group

- Vertical group

Ask patient to stand, and reinspect the venous pattern.

Varicose veins

S P E C I A L   T E C H N I Q U E S

EVALUATING ARTE-RIAL SUPPLY TO HAND. Feel ulnar pulse, if possible. Perform an **Allen test.** Ask patient to make a tight fist, palm up. Occlude both radial and ulnar arteries with your thumbs. Ask patient to open hand into a relaxed, slightly flexed position. Release your pressure over one artery. Palm should flush within about 3–5 seconds. Repeat, releasing other artery.

Persisting pallor of palm indicates occlusion of the released artery or its distal branches.

POSTURAL COLOR CHANGES OF CHRONIC ARTERIAL INSUFFICIENCY. Raise both legs to about 60° for about a minute Then ask

Marked pallor of feet on elevation, delayed color return and venous filling, and rubor of dependent feet suggest arterial insufficiency.

patient to sit up with legs dangling down. Note time required for (1) return of pinkness, normally about 10 seconds or less, and (2) filling of veins on feet and ankles, normally about 15 seconds. Watch for development of any unusual rubor.

THE MUSCULOSKELETAL SYSTEM

GENERAL APPROACH

Inspect the joints and surrounding tissues as you examine the various parts of the body.

Identify joints with changes in structure and function, carefully assessing affected joints for:

- Deformity or malalignment of bones

- Symmetry of involvement—one or both sides of the body; one joint or several

- Changes in surrounding soft tissue—skin changes, subcutaneous nodules, muscle atrophy, crepitus

- Limitations in range of motion, ligamentous laxity

Examination Techniques   **Possible Findings**

- Changes in muscle
  strength

Note signs of inflammation
and arthritis: swelling,
warmth, tenderness,
redness.

Outlined below are
examination techniques
appropriate to selected joints.

TEMPOROMANDIBULAR JOINT

Palpate the temporomandi-
bular joint as the patient
opens and closes the mouth.

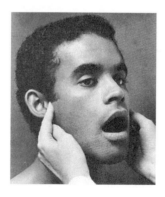

SHOULDERS

Inspect the contour of the
shoulders and shoulder
girdles from front and back.

Muscle atrophy anterior
or posterior dislocation
of humeral head

Examination Techniques	Possible Findings

Ask the patient to:

- Raise the arms to shoulder level, palms facing down

  Impaired glenohumeral motion

- Raise the arms vertically above the head, palms facing each other

  Impaired scapulothoracic motion (first 60°), impaired scapulothoracic and glenohumeral motion (final 30°)

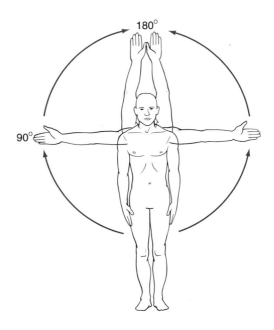

- Place both hands behind the neck, with elbows out (abduction and external rotation).

  Impaired external rotation of shoulder, as in arthritis, bursitis

Examination Techniques	Possible Findings
• Place both hands behind the small of the back (adduction and internal rotation).	Impaired internal rotation of shoulder, as in arthritis, bursitis

Assess areas of pain or tenderness.

• *Acromioclavicular joint:* Palpate, adduct arm across chest (crossover test).	Arthritis, inflammation
• *Subacromial and subdeltoid bursa:* Lift elbow posteriorly, palpate anterior to acromion and over sub-deltoid bursa.	Subacromial or subdeltoid bursitis

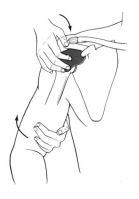

Rotator cuff: Lift elbow posteriorly, palpate head of humerus for tenderness over tendon insertions of "SITS" muscles (supraspinatus, infraspinatus,	Rotator cuff tendinitis

Examination Techniques   Possible Findings

teres minor; subscapularis
not palpable).

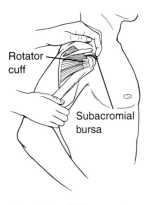

Check for ability to raise
arm to shoulder level
("drop arm" sign).

Inability to raise or
maintain arm at shoulder
level indicates rotator cuff
sprain or tear.

Bicipital groove and tendon:
Rotate humerus externally,
palpate bicipital groove;
alternatively, with forearm
flexed at right angle, supi-
nate forearm against
resistance.

Bicipital tenderness

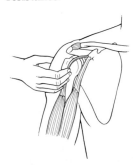

Examination Techniques	**Possible Findings**

ELBOWS

Inspect and palpate

- Olecranon process

  Olecranon bursitis; posterior dislocation from direct trauma or supra-condylar fracture

- Medial and lateral epicondyles

  Tender in epicondylitis

- Extensor surface of the ulnar

  Rheumatoid nodules

- Grooves overlying the elbow joint

  Tender in arthritis

Ask the patient to

- Flex and extend elbows

- Turn palms up and down (supination and pronation)

WRISTS AND HANDS

Inspect

- Movement of the wrist (flexion, extension, ulnar, and medial deviation), hands and fingers

  Guarded movement in injury

- Contours of wrists, hands, fingers

  Deformities in rheumatoid and degenerative arthritis; swelling in arthritis, ganglia; impaired alignment of fingers in flexor tendon damage

- Contours in palms

  Thenar atrophy in median nerve compression (carpal

Examination Techniques	**Possible Findings**

tunnel syndrome); hypothenar atrophy in ulnar nerve compression

Palpate

• Wrist joints

Wrist swelling in rheumatoid arthritis, gonococcal infection of joint or extensor tendon sheaths

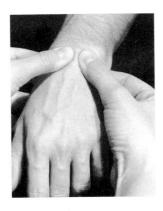

• Distal radius and ulna

Tenderness over ulnar styloid in Colles' fracture

• "Anatomic snuffbox"

Tenderness suggests scaphoid fracture

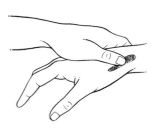

Examination Techniques	Possible Findings

- Metacarpophalangeal joint

Swelling in rheumatoid arthritis

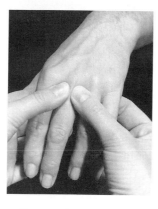

- Proximal and distal interphalangeal joint

Proximal nodules in rheumatoid arthritis (Bouchard's nodes), distal nodules in osteoarthritis (Heberden's nodes)

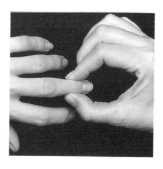

SPINE

Inspect spine from side and back, noting any abnormal

Kyphosis, scoliosis, lordosis, gibbus, list curvatures.

Examination Techniques	**Possible Findings**

Look for asymmetries
of shoulders, iliac crests,
or buttocks.

Pelvic tilt

Palpate

- Spinous processes of
  each vertebra

  Tender if trauma, infection

  "Step offs" in
  spondylolisthesis, fracture

- Sacroiliac joint

  Sacroiliitis

- Paravertebral muscles,
  if painful

  Paravertebral muscle spasm
  in abnormal posture,
  degenerative and
  inflammatory muscle
  processes

- Sciatic nerve

  Herniated disc nerve root
  compression

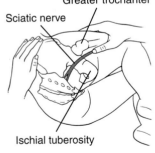

Greater trochanter

Sciatic nerve

Ischial tuberosity

Test the range of motion
in the neck and spine in

Decreased mobility in
arthritis

- Flexion

- Extension

Examination Techniques	Possible Findings

- Rotation

- Lateral bending

HIPS

Inspect gait for

- Stance (see below) and swing (foot moves forward, does not bear weight)

  Most problems appear during weight-bearing stance phase.

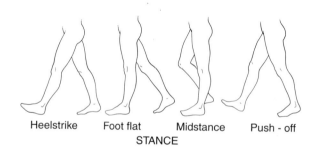

Heelstrike   Foot flat   Midstance   Push - off
STANCE

- Width of base (usually 2 to 4 inches from heel to heel) shift of pelvis, flexion of knee

  Cerebellar disease or foot problems in wide base

  Impaired shift of pelvis in arthritis, hip dislocation, abductor weakness

  Disrupted gait in lack of knee flexion

Examination Techniques   Possible Findings

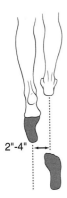

2"-4"

Palpate

- Along the inguinal ligament

  Bulges in inguinal hernia, aneurysm

- The *ileopectineal bursa,* lateral to the femoral pulse

  Tender in synovitis, bursitis, iliopsoas abscess

- The *trochanteric bursa,* on the greater trochanter of the femur

  Tender in trochanteric bursitis

- The *ischiogluteal bursa,* superficial to the ischeal tuberosity

  Tender in bursitis ("weaver's bottom")

Trochanteric Bursa

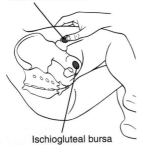

Ischiogluteal bursa

Examination Techniques   **Possible Findings**

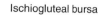

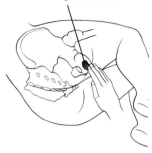

Ischiogluteal bursa

Check range of motion
including

• Flexion

Flexion of opposite leg
suggests deformity of that
hip.

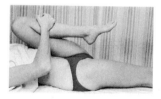

• Extension

Painful in iliopsoas abscess

• Abduction

Restricted in arthritis

Examination Techniques	Possible Findings

- Adduction

- Internal and external   Restricted in arthritis
  rotation

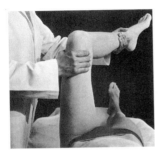

KNEES
Inspect

- Gait for knee extension   Stumbling or pushing knee
  at heel strike, flexion   into extension in
  during all other phases   quadriceps weakness
  of swing and stance

- Alignment of knees   Bowlegs, knockknees

- Contours of knees
  including

Inspect and palpate

- Patella   Swelling of prepatellar
                               bursitis ("housemaid's
                               knee")

- Suprapatellar pouch   Swelling in synovitis and
                               arthritis

Examination Techniques	Possible Findings

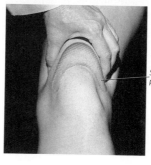

Suprapatellar pouch

- Infrapatellar spaces (hollow areas adjacent to patella)

  Swelling in arthritis

- Medial tibial condyle

  Swelling in *pes anserine* bursitis

- Popliteal surface

  Popliteal or "Baker's" cyst

Assess the patellofemoral compartment

- Palpate the patellar tendon and ask patient to extend the leg.

  Tenderness or inability to extend the leg in partial or complete tear of the patellar tendon

- Press the patella against the underlying femur.

  Pain, crepitus, and a history of knee pain suggest a patellofemoral disorder.

- Push patella distally and ask patient to tighten knee against table.

  Pain during contraction of quadriceps suggests *chondromalacia.*

With knees flexed, **palpate**

- Medial and lateral menisci

  Tenderness in medial or lateral meniscus tear

Examination Techniques	Possible Findings

- Medial collateral ligaments (MCLs) and lateral collateral ligaments (LCLs)

Tenderness in MCL or LCL sprain

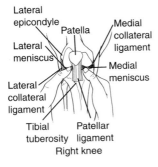

Assess any effusions

- The *Bulge Sign* for minor effusions: Compress the suprapatellar pouch, stroke downward on medial surface, apply pressure to force fluid to lateral surface, then tap knee behind lateral margin of patella.

A fluid wave returning to the medial surface after a lateral tap confirms an effusion—a positive "bulge sign."

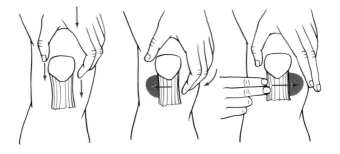

Examination Techniques	Possible Findings
• The *Balloon Sign* for major effusions: Compress the suprapatellar pouch with one hand and with thumb and finger of the other, feel for fluid entering the spaces next to the patella.	A palpable fluid wave is a positive sign.

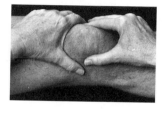

• *Ballotting the patella* for major effusions: Push the patella sharply against the femur; watch for fluid returning to the suprapatellar space.	Visible wave is a positive sign

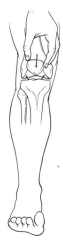

Examination Techniques   **Possible Findings**

If painful, **assess** ligaments.

- *Medial collateral ligament:*
  With knee slightly flexed,
  push medially against
  lateral surface of knee
  with one hand and pull
  laterally at the ankle with
  the other hand (an
  abduction or *valgus
  stress*).

Pain or a gap in the medial
joint line points to a partial
or complete MCL tear.

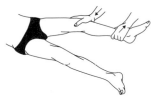

- *Lateral collateral
  ligament:* With knee
  slightly flexed, push
  laterally along medial
  surface of knee with
  one hand and pull
  medially at the ankle
  with the other hand
  (an *adduction* or *varus
  stress*).

Pain or a gap in the lateral
joint line points to a partial
or complete LCL tear (less
common than MCL
injuries).

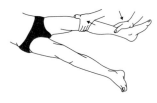

- *Anterior cruciate
  ligament:* With knee
  flexed, place thumbs on

If the proximal tibia slides
forward, there is a positive
anterior

Examination Techniques	Possible Findings

medial and lateral joint line and place fingers on hamstring insertions. Pull tibia forward and observe if it slides forward "like a drawer." Compare the degree of forward movement to that of the opposite knee.

drawer sign, and suggesting ACL ligamentous laxity or an ACL tear.

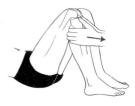

- Apply the *Lachman test:* Grasp the distal femur with one hand and the proximal tibia with the other (place the thumb on the joint line). Move the femur forward and the tibia back.

Significant forward excursion of the tibia suggests an ACL tear.

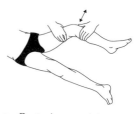

- *Posterior cruciate ligament:* Position the patient and examining hands as described in the ACL test. Push the tibia posteriorly and observe for posterior movement.

Isolated PCL tears are rare.

Examination Techniques   Possible Findings

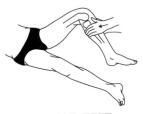

ANKLES AND FEET

Inspect ankles and feet.   Hallux valgus, corns,
                                      calluses

Palpate

• Ankle joint and ligaments   Tender joint in arthritis,
                               tender ligaments in sprain

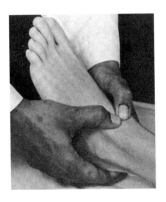

• Achilles tendon   Rheumatoid nodules,
                               tenderness in tendinitis

• **Compress** the metatarso- Tenderness in arthritis and
  phalangeal joints; then   other conditions
  palpate each joint
  between the thumb and
  forefinger.

Examination Techniques   **Possible Findings**

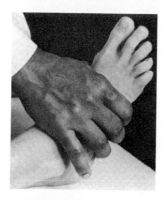

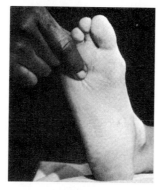

Assess range of motion

- Dorsiflex and plantar flex the ankle (*tibiotalar joint*).

  An arthritic joint often hurts when moved in any direction. A sprain hurts chiefly when the injured ligament is stretched.

- Stabilize the ankle and invert and evert the heel (*subtalar* or *talocalcaneal joint*).

  Ankle sprain

Examination Techniques   Possible Findings

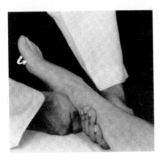

INVERSION

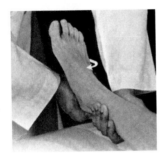

EVERSION

- Stabilize the heel and   Trauma, arthritis
  invert and evert the
  forefoot (*transverse
  tarsal joints*).

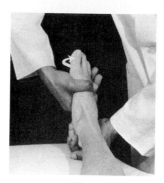

INVERSION

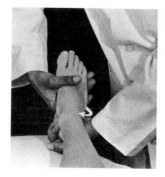

EVERSION

- Flex toes at *metatarso-phalangeal joints*.

Examination Techniques   Possible Findings

S P E C I A L   M A N E U V E R S

PHALEN'S TEST FOR CARPAL TUNNEL SYNDROME. Hold patient's wrists in acute flexion, or ask patient to press backs of both hands together to form right angles. Either position should be held for 60 seconds.

Numbness or tingling over distribution of median nerve is a positive sign, suggesting carpal tunnel syndrome.

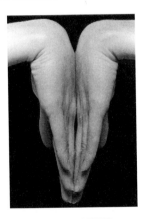

PHALEN'S TEST

TINEL'S SIGN FOR CARPAL TUNNEL SYNDROME. Percuss lightly over median nerve at wrist.

Tingling or electric sensations in distribution of median nerve is a positive sign.

Examination Techniques   Possible Findings

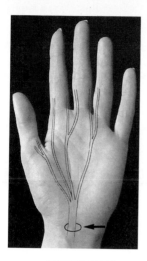

TINEL'S SIGN

○— STRAIGHT LEG RAIS-
ING. Raise patient's straight-
ened leg until pain occurs.
Then dorsiflex foot.

Sharp pain down back of
leg suggests tension on or
compression of a nerve
root. Dorsiflexion increases
pain.

○— MEASURING LEG
LENGTH. Patient's legs
should be aligned symmet-
rically. With a tape,
measure distance from an-
terior superior iliac spine to
medial malleolus. Tape
should cross knee medially.

Unequal leg length may be
the cause of scoliosis.

↳/○— MEASURING
RANGE OF MOTION. To
measure range of motion
precisely, a simple pocket
goniometer is needed.
Estimates may be made

A flexion deformity of 45°
and further flexion to 90°
(45° → 90°).

Examination Techniques   **Possible Findings**

visually. Movement in the
elbow at the right is limited
to range indicated by red
lines.

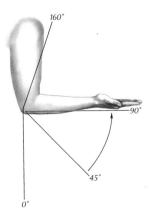

THE NERVOUS SYSTEM

MENTAL STATUS

Recall what you know
about the patient's mental
status as it relates to the
nervous system, and **assess**
it further if indicated.

CRANIAL NERVES

CN 1 (OLFACTORY). **Test**   Loss in frontal lobe lesions
sense of smell on each side.

CN II (OPTIC)
Assess visual acuity.   Blindness
Check visual fields.   Hemianopsia

Examination Techniques	**Possible Findings**

Inspect optic discs.

Papilledema, optic atrophy

CN II, III (OPTIC AND OCULOMOTOR). **Test** pupillary reactions to light. If they are abnormal, test reactions to near effort.

Blindness, CN III paralysis, tonic pupils, Horner's syndrome may affect light reactions

CN III, IV, VI (OCULO-MOTOR, TROCHLEAR, AND ABDUCENS). **Assess** extraocular movements.

Strabismus from paralysis of CN III, IV, or VI; nystagmus

CN V (TRIGEMINAL) **Feel** the contractions of temporal and masseter muscles.

Motor or sensory loss from lesions of CN V or its higher motor pathways

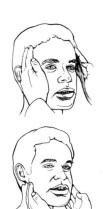

Check corneal reflexes.

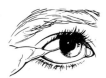

Examination Techniques	Possible Findings

Test pain and light touch sensations on face.

CN VII (FACIAL). **Ask** patient to raise both eyebrows, frown, close eyes tightly, show teeth, smile, and puff out cheeks.

Weakness from lesion of peripheral nerve, as in Bell's palsy, or of central nervous system, as in a stroke

CN VIII (ACOUSTIC). **Assess** hearing. If it is decreased—

• Test for lateralization (**Weber test**).

Sensorineural loss causes lateralization to less affected ear and AC > BC. Conduction loss causes lateralization to more affected ear and BC > AC.

• Compare air and bone conduction (**Rinne test**).

CN IX, X (GLOSSOPHARYNGEAL AND VAGUS)

Observe any difficulty in swallowing.

A weakened palate or pharynx impairs swallowing.

Listen to the voice.

Hoarse or nasal voice

Watch soft palate rise with "ah."

Palatal paralysis

Test gag reflex on each side.

Absent reflex

CN XI (SPINAL ACCESSORY)

• *Trapezius muscles.* **Assess** muscles for bulk, involuntary movements, and strength of shoulder shrug.

Atrophy, fasciculations, weakness

Examination Techniques	Possible Findings
• *Sternomastoid muscles:* **Assess** strength as head turns against your hand.	Weakness

CN XII (HYPOGLOSSAL)

Listen to patient's articulation.	Dysarthria from damage to CN X or CN XII
Inspect the resting tongue.	Atrophy, fasciculations
Inspect the protruded tongue.	Deviation to weak side

℞ THE MOTOR SYSTEM

BODY POSITION	Hemiplegia in stroke
INVOLUNTARY MOVEMENTS. If movements are present, **observe** their location, quality, rate, rhythm, amplitude, and setting.	Tremors, fasciculations, tics, chorea, athetosis, oral–facial dyskinesias
MUSCLE BULK. **Inspect** muscle contours.	Atrophy
MUSCLE TONE. **Assess** resistance to passive stretch of arms and legs.	Spasticity, rigidity, flaccidity
MUSCLE STRENGTH in major muscle groups:	

Examination Techniques   Possible Findings

TABLE 3-1 MUSCLE STRENGTH GRADING SCALE

Grade	Description
0	No muscular contraction detected
1	A barely detectable trace of contraction
2	Active movement with gravity eliminated
3	Active movement against gravity
4	Active movement against gravity and some resistance
5	Active movement against full resistance

- Elbow flexion (C5, C6)

- Elbow extension (C6, C7, C8)

- Wrist extension (C6, C7, C8, radial nerve)

- Grip (C7, C8, T1)

- Finger abduction (C8, T1, ulnar nerve)

Look for a pattern in any detectable weakness. It may suggest a lower motor neuron lesion affecting a peripheral nerve or nerve root. Weakness of one side of body suggests an upper motor neuron lesion. A polyneuropathy causes symmetrical distal weakness, and a myopathy usually causes proximal weakness. Weakness that worsens with repeated effort and improves with rest suggests myasthenia gravis.

Examination Techniques Possible Findings

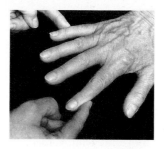

- Thumb opposition
  (C8, T1, median nerve)

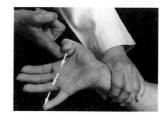

- Trunk—flexion,
  extension, lateral
  bending

- Hip flexion (L2, L3,
  L4)

- Hip adduction
  (L2, L3, L4)

- Hip abduction
  (L4, L5, S1)

- Hip extension (S1)

- Knee extension
  (L2, L3, L4)

Examination Techniques	Possible Findings

- Knee flexion (L4, L5, S1, S2)

- Ankle dorsiflexion (L4, L5)

- Ankle plantar flexion (S1)

COORDINATION. **Check:**

Rapid alternating movements in arms and legs	Clumsy, slow movements in cerebellar disease
Point-to-point movements in arms and legs	Clumsy, unsteady movements in cerebellar disease

⌇   *Gait.* **Ask** patient to

- Walk away, turn, and come back

    Upper or lower motor neuron weakness, cere-bellar ataxia, parkinsonism, and loss of position sense may all affect performance.

- Walk heel-to-toe

- Walk on toes, then on heels

- Hop in place on each foot

- Do one-legged shallow knee bends

(Substitute rising from a chair and climbing on a stool for hops and bends as indicated.)

Stance

- **Do** a *Romberg test* (a sensory test of stance).

    Loss of balance that appears when eyes are

Examination Techniques	Possible Findings

Ask patient to stand with feet together and eyes open, then closed for 20–30 seconds. Mild swaying may occur. (Stand close by to prevent falls.)

closed is a positive Romberg test, suggesting poor position sense.

- **Look** for a *pronator drift.* Watch as patient holds arms forward, with eyes closed, for 20–30 seconds.

Flexion and pronation at elbow and downward drift of arm in hemiplegia

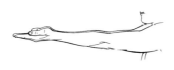

Ask patient to keep arms up, and **tap** them downward. A smooth return to position is normal.

Weakness, incoordination, poor position sense

THE SENSORY SYSTEM

METHODS OF TESTING

Compare symmetrical areas on the two sides of the body.

Hemisensory deficits

Also **compare** distal and proximal areas of arms and legs for *pain, temperature,* and *touch sensation.* Scatter stimuli to sample most dermatomes and major peripheral nerves.

Glove-and-stocking loss of peripheral neuropathy

Examination Techniques	Possible Findings
Check fingers and toes distally for *vibration and position senses.* If responses are abnormal, test more proximally.	Loss of position and vibration senses in posterior column disease
Map any area of abnormal response.	
Except when you are explaining the tests, patient's eyes should be closed.	
Assess response to the following stimuli:	
• *Pain.* Use the sharp end of a pin or other suitable tool. The dull end serves as a control.	Analgesia, hypalgesia, hyperalgesia
• *Temperature* (if indicated). Use test tubes with hot and ice-cold water (or other objects of suitable temperature).	Temperature and pain senses usually correlate with each other.
• *Light touch.* Use a fine wisp of cotton.	Anesthesia, hyperesthesia
• *Vibration.* Use a 128-Hz or 256-Hz tuning fork, held on a bony prominence.	Vibration and position senses, both carried in the posterior columns, often correlate with each other.

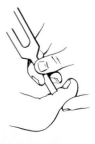

Examination Techniques   **Possible Findings**

- *Position.* Holding
  patient's finger or big
  toe by its sides, move it
  up or down.

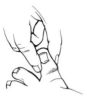

Also **assess** one or more of
the *discriminative* sensations:

- *Stereognosis.* Ask for
  identification of a
  common object placed
  in patient's hand.

  Stereognosis, number
  identification, and two-
  point discrimination may
  be impaired by lesions in
  the posterior columns or in
  the sensory cortex.

- *Number identification.*
  Ask for identification of
  a number drawn on
  patient's palm with blunt
  end of a pen.

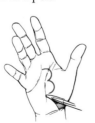

- *Two-point discrimination.*
  Find minimal distance
  on pad of patient's
  finger at which the sides

Examination Techniques   **Possible Findings**

of two points can be
distinguished from one
(normally <5 mm).

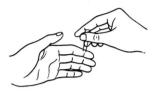

- *Point localization.* Touch
skin briefly, and ask
patient to open both
eyes and identify the
place touched.

A lesion in the sensory
cortex may impair point
localization on the opposite
side and cause extinction
of the touch sensation on
that side.

- *Extinction.* Simulta-
neously touch opposite,
corresponding areas of
the body, and ask patient
where the touch is felt.

ϑ/o—   **REFLEXES**

TABLE 3-2 REFLEX GRADING SCALE

Grade	Description
4+	Hyperactive (with clonus)
3+	Brisker than average, not necessarily abnormal
2+	**Average, normal**
1+	Diminished, low normal
0	No response

Examination Techniques   **Possible Findings**

• Biceps (C5, C6)

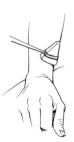

Hyperactive deep tendon
reflexes, absent abdominal
reflexes, and a Babinski
response indicate an upper
motor neuron lesion.

• Triceps (C6, C7)

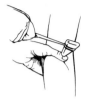

• Supinator (brachio-
radialis) (C5, C6)

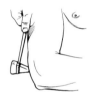

o— • Abdominals

Abdominal reflexes may be
absent with upper or lower
neuron lesions.

Examination Techniques   Possible Findings

Upper (T8, T9, T10)

Lower (T10, T11, T12)

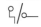 • Knee (L2, L3, L4)

 • Ankle (S1)   Ankle jerks symmetrically
                                decreased or absent in
                                peripheral polyneuropathy

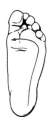

 • Plantar (L5, S1),   Babinski response
   normally flexor

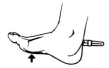   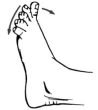

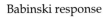

Examination Techniques   **Possible Findings**

Check for clonus if
reflexes seem hyperactive

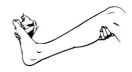

Reinforce absent reflexes
by isometric contraction
of unrelated muscles.

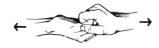

S P E C I A L   T E C H N I Q U E S

WINGING. Ask pa-
tient to push against the
wall or your hand with a
partially straightened arm.
Inspect the scapula. It should
stay close to the chest wall.

Winging of scapula away
from the chest wall
suggests weakness of the
serratus anterior muscle.

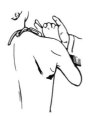

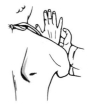

ANAL REFLEX. With
a dull object, stroke
outward from anus in four
quadrants.Watch for anal
contraction.

Loss of reflex suggests
lesion at S 2-3-4 level.

Examination Techniques   **Possible Findings**

ASTERIXIS. Ask the patient to hold both arms forward, with hands cocked up and fingers spread. Watch for 1–2 minutes.

Sudden brief flexions suggest a metabolic encephalopathy.

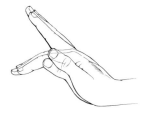

MENINGEAL SIGNS. With patient supine, flex head and neck toward chest. Note resistance or pain, and watch for flexion of hips and knees (**Brudzinski's sign**).

Meningeal irritation may cause resistance to and pain on flexion during both these maneuvers.

Flex one of patient's legs at hip and knee, then straighten knee. Note resistance or pain (**Kernig's sign**).

A compressed lumbosacral nerve root also causes pain on straightening the knee of a raised leg.

ASSESSING THE STUPOROUS OR COMATOSE PATIENT. **Assess** ABCs (airway, breathing, and circulation).

Take pulse, blood pressure, and rectal temperature.

Establish level of consciousness with escalating stimuli.

Lethargy, obtundation, stupor, coma

Examination Techniques	Possible Findings

Don't dilate pupils, and **don't flex** patient's neck if cervical cord may have been injured.

Observe

- Breathing pattern

  Cheyne–Stokes, ataxic breathing

- Pupils

  Pinpoint, midposition, one dilated and fixed

- Ocular movements

  Deviation to one side

Note posture of body.

Decorticate rigidity, decerebrate rigidity, flaccid hemiplegia

Test for flaccid paralysis.

- Hold the forearms vertically and note wrist positions.

  A flaccid hand droops to the horizontal.

- From 12–18 inches above bed, drop each arm.

  A flaccid arm drops more rapidly.

- Support both knees in a somewhat flexed position, and then extend each knee and let lower leg drop to the bed.

  The flaccid leg drops more rapidly.

- From a similar starting position, release both legs.

  A flaccid leg falls into extension and external rotation.

Check for the *oculocephalic reflex (doll's-eye movements)*. Holding upper eyelids open, turn head quickly to each side, then flex and extend patient's

In a comatose patient with an intact brainstem, the eyes move in the opposite direction, in this case to her left (doll's-eye movements).

Examination Techniques   **Possible Findings**

neck. This patient's head
will be turned to her right.

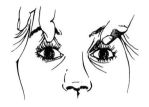 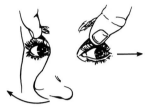

Very deep coma or a lesion
in midbrain or pons
abolishes this reflex.

Complete the neurologic
and general physical
examination.

4

THE PHYSICAL EXAMINATION OF INFANTS AND CHILDREN

OVERVIEW

While most of the techniques used to examine adults are applicable to infants and children, some methods of examination are unique during infancy (the first year of life), early childhood (1–4 years), and late childhood (5–12 years). When there are differences in technique, they will be described here, following the outline for each of the sections of Chapter 3, The Physical Examination of an Adult. Where no differences exist, no comment will be made. The physical examination of adolescents (13–20 years) essentially conforms to that of the adult.

Recommendations for Preventive Pediatric Health Care appear on pp. 130–132.

SEQUENCE OF A COMPREHENSIVE EXAMINATION

Positions for various parts of the examination during infancy and early childhood do not necessarily follow those recommended for examining adults. Some parts can be conducted on the parent's or your lap with the baby supine or sitting. The supine position on the examining table is essential for examination of the abdomen, hips, genitalia, and rectum, and also of the mouth and the ears when the baby is resisting.

Examination Techniques   Possible Findings

Infancy and Early Childhood.
No special sequence except
that oral and ear examination, abduction of the hips,
and the rectal examination
(if needed) should be saved
until last, since these usually cause the baby to cry.
Be astute and listen to the
heart and lungs and palpate
the abdomen when the baby
is quiet.

Late Childhood. Use the
same order of examination
as with adults, except
examine the most painful
areas last.

MENTAL AND PHYSICAL STATUS

Infancy. **Observe** the parents' affect in talking about
their baby, their manner of
holding, moving, and
dressing the baby, and their
response to situations that
may produce discomfort
for the baby. **Observe** a
breast or bottle feeding.

Normal parental bonding
to the infant. Maladaptive
parental nurturing as a
cause of malnutrition and
"failure to thrive"

Determine attainment of
developmental milestones
using the Denver Develop-
mental Screening Test be-
fore conducting the physical examination.

Normal development
versus delays in personal-
social, fine motor-adaptive,
language, and gross motor
development

Early Childhood. **Observe**
during the interview the degree of sickness or wellness,

Normal or abnormal level
of general health and
development. Parents who

Examination Techniques	Possible Findings

mood, state of nutrition, speech, cry, facial expression, apparent chronological and emotional age, developmental skills, and parent-child interaction, including the amount of separation tolerance, displays of affection, and response to discipline.

abuse their children often pay little attention to them; abused children usually demonstrate no anxiety when separated from their parents.

Late Childhood. **Determine** the child's orientation to time and place, factual knowledge, and language and number skills. **Observe** motor skills used in writing, tying shoelaces, buttoning, using scissors, and drawing.

Normal or abnormal performance, the latter suggesting intellectual impairment or motor disability

THE GENERAL SURVEY

Measurements of vital signs and body size in infants and children often provide the first and only indicators of disease.

Sepsis, chronic renal failure, congenital heart disease, parental deprivation

HEIGHT AND WEIGHT

Growth, reflected in increases in body height and weight within expected limits, is probably the best indicator of health during infancy and childhood. **Plot** each child's height and weight on standard growth charts to determine if normal progress is being made. See standard grids on pp. 142–145.

Growth measures above the 97th or below the 3rd percentile, or if there has been a recent rise or fall from prior levels, require investigation.

Examination Techniques	Possible Findings

HEAD CIRCUMFERENCE

Determine the head circumference at every physical examination during the first 2 years. See standard grids on pp. 146–147.

Microcephaly, premature closure of the sutures, hydrocephalus, subdural hematoma, brain tumor

With the patient supine, **place** a cloth, soft plastic, or disposable paper centimeter tape over the occipital, parietal, and frontal prominences of the head.

Individual and/or serial measurements of the head circumference are essential for determination of retarded and overly rapid growth of the head.

Stretch the tape and **note** the reading, being sure that the greatest circumference is obtained.

S P E C I A L   T E C H N I Q U E

FLUSH TECHNIQUE FOR MEASURING BLOOD PRESSURE (in infants and children <3 years of age). With cuff in place, wrap an elastic bandage snugly around the elevated arm, proceeding from fingers to antecubital space. Inflate cuff to a pressure above the expected systolic reading.

Remove bandage and place the pallid arm at patient's side. Allow pressure to fall slowly until flush of color returns to forearm, hand, and fingers.

When flushing occurs, the sphygmomanometer reading will indicate a blood pressure value somewhere between systolic and diastolic levels.

Examination Techniques	**Possible Findings**

THE SKIN

Infancy. **Look** for

- Pallor

    Anoxia, anemia

- Vasomotor changes

    Mottled appearance common in prematurity, cretinism, Down's syndrome

- Cyanosis

    Acrocyanosis, congenital heart disease

- Melanotic pigmentation

    Mongolian spots

- Jaundice

    Sepsis, hemolytic disease, biliary obstruction

- Erythema

    Miliaria rubra, erythema toxicum, capillary hemangioma, port-wine stain

THE HEAD

Infancy. **Palpate** the

    Head small with microcephaly, enlarged with hydrocephaly

- Anterior and posterior fontanelles

    Fontanelles full and tense with meningitis

- Sagittal, coronal, and lambdoidal sutures

    Closed with microcephaly. Separated with increased intracranial pressure (hydrocephaly, subdural hematoma, and brain tumor)

- Cranial bones

    Swelling due to subperiosteal hemorrhage

Examination Techniques	Possible Findings

(cephalohematoma) does not cross suture lines; swelling due to bleeding associated with a fracture does.

Early and Late Childhood. **Auscultate** the skull.

A bruit in a nonanemic child suggests increased intracranial pressure or an intracranial arteriovenous shunt.

SPECIAL TECHNIQUES

MACEWEN's SIGN. Percuss the parietal bone on each side by tapping your index or middle finger directly against its surface.

A "cracked pot" sound is heard prior to closure of the sutures and when increased intracranial pressure causes closed sutures to separate (e.g., in lead encephalopathy and brain tumor).

TRANSILLUMINATION OF THE SKULL. In a completely darkened room, place a standard three-battery flashlight, with a soft rubber collar attached to the lighted end, flush against the skull at various points. Normally, a 2-cm halo of light is present around the circumference of the flashlight over the frontoparietal area, and a 1-cm halo over the occipital area.

Uniform transillumination of the entire head occurs when the cerebral cortex is partially absent or thinned. Localized bright spots may be seen with subdural effusion and porencephalic cysts.

CHVOSTEK'S SIGN. Percuss the top of the cheek just below the zygomatic

One or two contractions of the facial muscles may occur normally during

Examination Techniques	Possible Findings

bone in front of the ear, using the tip of your index or middle finger.

infancy and early childhood. Repeated contractions occur in tetanus and in tetany due to hypocalcemia and hyperventilation.

THE EYES

Infancy. **Test** for vision by shining a bright light into the eye or moving an object quickly toward it.

Blinking of the eyes and extension of the head will occur if the baby can see.

Early and Late Childhood. **Test** vision of children over age 3 years with the Snellen E chart. Most youngsters will indicate the direction of the E, either orally or by pointing. Normal visual acuity is about 20/40 at age 3 years, 20/30 at age 4 years, and 20/20 at age 6–7 years.

Any difference in visual acuity between the eyes (e.g., 20/20 on left and 20/30 on right) is abnormal, might lead to amblyopia, and should be referred to an ophthalmologist.

SPECIAL TECHNIQUE

EXAMINATION OF AN INFANT'S EYES. Hold the baby upright, grasping the axillae with your hands and fixing the head with your thumbs. Extend your arms and rotate yourself with the baby slowly in one direction. The baby's eyes will open, providing a clear view of the scleras, irises, and extraocular movements.

The eyes look in the direction you are turning. When the rotation stops, the eyes look in the opposite direction.

| Examination Techniques | Possible Findings |

THE EARS

THE AURICLE

Infancy. **Note** whether the upper portion of the newborn's auricle joins the scalp below a line drawn across the inner canthus and outer canthus of the eye.

Auricles that join the scalp below this line suggest the presence of renal agenesis.

THE EAR CANAL AND EARDRUM

Infancy. **Look** at the eardrum with your otoscope by pulling the pinna downward.

The light reflex on the tympanic membrane is diffuse and does not become cone-shaped until several months after birth.

HEARING

Infancy. **Make** a loud, sharp noise near the infant's ear and **watch** for blinking of the eyes (**acoustic blink reflex**).

Absence may indicate decreased hearing.

S P E C I A L   T E C H N I Q U E

PNEUMATIC OTOSCOPY. Place the speculum of a pneumatic otoscope far enough into the external ear canal to provide a relatively tight air seal. Introduce or remove air from the canal by applying positive and negative pressures with a rubber squeeze bulb attached to the otoscope.

When air is introduced the tympanic membrane moves inward, and when air is removed the membrane moves outward. This movement is absent in serous otitis media, and diminished in some cases of acute otitis media.

Examination Techniques	Possible Findings

THE NOSE, MOUTH, PHARYNX, AND NECK

NOSE

Infancy. **Test** patency of the nasal passages by occluding each nostril alternately while holding infant's mouth closed.

The baby will be unable to breathe when choanal atresia is present.

MOUTH

Early and Late Childhood. **Ask** child to bite down as hard as possible. **Part** the lips and **observe** alignment of maxilla and mandible.

Normally, the upper teeth slightly override the lower teeth. Overbite and underbite can be detected this way.

PHARYNX

Examine the throat. **Note** size and appearance of tonsils. They are relatively larger in early and late childhood than in infancy and adolescence. They usually have deep crypts on their surfaces, often with white concretions or food particles protruding from their depths—no indication of current or past disease.

A white exudate on the tonsils suggests strepto-coccal tonsillitis. A thick, gray, adherent exudate suggests diphtheritic tonsillitis. Necrosis (grayish discoloration of the tissue itself) suggests infectious mononucleosis. One red tonsil protruding forward and medially strongly indicates a peritonsillar abscess.

NECK

Infancy. **Inspect** and **palpate** the newborn's neck for skin tags, fistulas, masses, cysts, muscle spasm, and crepitus.

Thyroglossal duct fistula or cyst, branchial cleft fistula or cyst, and sternomastoid muscle injury and fractured clavicle from birth trauma

Examination Techniques	Possible Findings

THE THORAX AND LUNGS

Infancy

- **Note** the breathing pattern.

Alternating rapid (30–40/min) and slow (5–10/min) respirations are considered normal ("periodic") breathing. Apnea (>20 sec) with cardiopulmonary or CNS disease or with high risk for sudden infant death syndrome (SIDS)

- **Note** head movement with breathing.

Extension of head on inspiration with severe respiratory disease

Auscultate the chest with the bell or small diaphragm, listening for breath sounds.

Rarely absent, even with atelectasis, effusion, empyema, or pneumothorax. Inspiratory wheeze with narrowing of upper airway, expiratory wheeze with narrowing of lower airway. Fine crackles normally heard at the end of deep inspiration

THE BREASTS

BREASTS

Infancy. **Look** for enlargement of the newborn's breasts with white discharge from nipples.

Normal maternal estrogenic effect lasting several days

Late Childhood. **Look** for asymmetry of breast size in females.

Usual during pre-adolescence

Examination Techniques	Possible Findings

THE CARDIOVASCULAR SYSTEM

THE ARTERIAL PULSE

Palpate the femoral pulses.

Diminution (as compared to radial pulse) or absence with coarctation of the aorta

BLOOD PRESSURE

For measurement of blood pressure in children under 3 years of age, see the flush method, page 114. For normal and abnormal levels of blood pressure in children, see pp. 192–198.

THE HEART

Look and **palpate** for the apical pulse.

At 4th interspace until age 7 years, at 5th interspace thereafter. To left of mid-clavicular line until age 4 years, at MCL ages 4 to 6 years, and to right of MCL after age 7 years.

THE ABDOMEN

Infancy. **Inspect** the new-born's umbilical cord.

There should be two thick-walled arteries and one thin-walled vein. A single umbilical artery suggests the presence of a variety of congenital anomalies.

Examination Techniques	Possible Findings

SPECIAL TECHNIQUES

EXAMINATION FOR PY-LORIC STENOSIS. Place un-clothed infant supine and stand at foot of examining table. Direct a bright light at table height across the abdomen from infant's right side. Feed baby a bottle of sugar water and observe abdomen closely.

With pyloric stenosis, peristaltic waves are seen going across the upper abdomen from left to right with increasing amplitude and frequency until infant vomits with projectile force.

After vomiting occurs, pal-pate deeply in right upper quadrant with baby supine and then prone, using your extended middle finger.

The hypertrophied pyloric muscle about 2 cm in diameter will be felt.

SCRATCH TEST TO DETER-MINE LIVER SIZE. Place di-aphragm of stethoscope just above right costal margin at midclavicular line. With your fingernail, lightly scratch skin of abdomen along the midclavicular line, moving from below umbili-cus toward costal margin. Listen for the scratching sound.

When the fingernail reaches the liver's lower edge, the sound of scratching will first be heard as it is transmitted through the liver.

MALE GENITALIA

HERNIAS

Early and Late Childhood.
Ask the child to try to lift the chair in which you are sitting.

This will help you to detect inguinal and femoral hernias not discovered when the child was asked to cough or strain down.

Examination Techniques	Possible Findings

S P E C I A L   T E C H N I Q U E

DETECTION OF PSEUDO-UNDESCENDED TESTICLE. Because the cremasteric reflex is so strong during early and late childhood, you may not be able to feel a testicle while examining the scrotum with the child upright or supine. To check for a truly undescended testicle, sit the child cross-legged and palpate the inguinal canal and scrotum.

This positioning interrupts the cremasteric reflex and allows the testicle to descend into the scrotum.

FEMALE GENITALIA

Examine the *female genitalia* while the patient is in the supine frog-leg position. Separate the labia majora at their midpoint with the thumb of each hand applying traction laterally and posteriorly. Inspect the *urethral orifice* and the *vestibule,* defined by the labia minora laterally, the clitoris anteriorly, and the posterior fourchette. Look for the *hymen,* a thickened, avascular structure with a central orifice that covers the vaginal opening.

Enlargement of clitoris and posterior fusion of labia majora are signs of *ambiguous genitalia.* When present, it is essential to determine the sex of the child before a definite sex assignment is made.

Fusion of labia minora is seen occasionally in girls under 4 years of age. It may be partial, with only the posterior portion of the labia fused, or it may be complete. A thin membrane that joins the labial edges is easily lysed with a cotton swab.

Examination Techniques	Possible Findings

THE MUSCULOSKELETAL SYSTEM

Screening the Child's Musculoskeletal System

Observe the child

• Standing upright with feet together	Foot deformities, bow legs, knock-knees, scoliosis
• Walking and running	Limp and other gait abnormalities due to muscle weakness or spasticity
• Stooping to pick up an object	Eye–hand coordination and muscle balance
• Rising from a supine position on the floor	General neurologic integrity and the proximal leg muscle weakness of muscular dystrophy (**Gower's sign**)

THE SPINE

Inspect and **palpate** the lumbosacral spine carefully.

• **Look** and **feel** for defects of the vertebral bodies.	Defects (spina bifida occulta) may be associated with an underlying spinal cord anomaly (diastematomyelia).
• **Look** for abnormalities of the skin, pigmented	A sinus tract provides potential entry to the spinal

Examination Techniques	Possible Findings

spots, hair patches, or deep pits that might overlie external openings of sinus tracts that extend to the spinal canal.

canal of organisms that can cause meningitis.

SPECIAL TECHNIQUES

ORTOLANI TEST. With infant supine, legs pointing toward you, flex legs to 90° at hips and knees. Place your index fingers over the greater trochanters of the femurs and your thumbs over the lesser trochanters. Abduct both hips simultaneously until the lateral aspect of each knee touches examining table.

When a congenitally dislocated hip is present in a newborn, a click is heard or felt as the femoral head enters the acetabulum near the end of abduction (**Ortolani's sign**). In older infants, decreased abduction of the affected hip(s) may be the only finding of dislocation.

TRENDELENBURG TEST. Observe patient from behind as weight is shifted from one leg to the other.

Note if the pelvis remains level (**negative Trendelenburg sign**) or tilts toward the opposite side (**positive sign**).

A positive Trendelenburg sign is present in diseases of the hip associated with gluteus medius muscle weakness.

THE NERVOUS SYSTEM

REFLEXES

Infancy. Because the corticospinal pathways are not fully developed at birth, the spinal reflex mechanisms are variable during infancy.

Examination Techniques	Possible Findings

- *Triceps*—Usually not present until after 6 months

- *Abdominals*—Absent at birth, but appear within 6 months

- *Ankle*—Unsustained ankle clonus (8–10 beats) is normal.

  Sustained ankle clonus suggests severe CNS disease.

- *Plantar*—Babinski response present in some (<10%) normal newborns and may remain for as long as 2 years

INFANTILE AUTOMATISMS

Specific reflex activities that test brainstem and spinal cord functions are found in newborns and disappear in early infancy.

Presence or absence of these reflexes does not predict immediate or eventual cortical function positively or negatively. However, absence in the newborn or their persistence beyond their expected time of disappearance suggests severe CNS disease.

PALMAR GRASP REFLEX— disappears at 3 to 4 months

With baby's head in the midline position and arms semiflexed, **place** your index fingers from the ulnar side into baby's hands and **press** against palmar surfaces.

The baby responds by flexing all of its fingers to grasp your fingers.

Examination Techniques	Possible Findings
ROOTING REFLEX— disappears at 3 to 4 months; may be present longer during sleep	
With baby's head in the midline position and hands resting on the anterior chest, **stroke** with your forefinger skin at corners of mouth.	Mouth opens and the head turns to the stroked side.
Stroke middle of upper lip.	Mouth opens and head extends.
Stroke middle of lower lip.	Mouth opens and chin drops.
TRUNK INCURVATION (GALANT'S) REFLEX—disappears at 2 months	
Suspend baby prone in one of your hands.	
Stimulate one side of the baby's back approximately 1 cm from the midline along a paravertebral line extending from shoulders to buttocks.	The trunk curves toward the stimulated side with movement of shoulders and pelvis in that direction.
VERTICAL SUSPENSION POSITIONING—disappears after 4 months	
Hold baby upright facing away from you with your hands under the axillae.	Normally, head is maintained in the midline and legs flex at hips and knees. Fixed extension and crossed adduction of the legs (scissoring) indicate spastic paraplegia or diplegia.

Examination Techniques	Possible Findings

PLACING RESPONSE—best
after 4 days; disappearance
time variable

Hold baby upright facing
away from you with your
hands under the axillae and
your thumbs supporting
back of head.

Allow dorsal surface of one
foot to touch the undersurface of a table top, taking
care not to plantar flex
the foot. **Repeat** process
with other foot.

The foot is lifted reflexly
and placed on the table top.

Once both feet are placed
on the table top, **propel** the
baby forward slowly.

A series of alternate step-
ping movements of legs
and feet occurs.

ROTATION TEST—disappear-
ance time variable

Hold baby upright facing
you with your hands under
the arms. **Turn** yourself
around in one direction and
then the other.

Baby's head turns in
direction in which you
turn.

Restrain baby's head with
your thumbs as you turn.

Baby's eyes turn in
direction in which you
turn.

TONIC NECK REFLEX—may
be present at birth, but usually appears at 2 months
and disappears at 6 months

With baby supine, **turn** its
head to one side and **hold**
its chin over its shoulder.

Arm and leg on side to
which head is turned ex-
tend, while other arm and

Examination Techniques	Possible Findings
Repeat the maneuver, turning the head to the opposite side.	leg flex. The reflex is considered abnormal when it occurs every time it is evoked.
PEREZ REFLEX—disappears after 3 months	
Suspend baby prone in one of your hands. **Press** the thumb of your other hand over the sacrum and **move** it firmly over the spine upward to the neck.	Head and spine extend, knees flex on the abdomen, and baby cries and urinates.
MORO RESPONSE OR STARTLE REFLEX—disappears by 4 months	
Hold baby in the supine position, supporting head, back, and legs. Then suddenly **lower** the entire body about 2 feet and **stop** abruptly; or—	Arms abduct briskly and extend at elbows with hands open and fingers extended; legs flex slightly and abduct, but less so than the arms. Arms then come forward over body in a clasping movement, and simultaneously baby cries.
Produce a loud noise (e.g., strike examining table with palms of your hands on both sides of baby's head).	

RECOMMENDATIONS FOR PREVENTIVE PEDIATRIC CARE

Each child and family is unique; therefore, these Recommendations are designed for healthy children with competent parenting and satisfactory growth and development. Additional visits may become necessary when circumstances vary from normal.

Infancy

AGE	2–4 days[1]	By 1 mo	2 mo	4 mo	6 mo	8 mo	10 mo	12 mo
HISTORY Initial/Interval	•	•	•	•	•	•	•	•
MEASURE-MENTS								
Height and Weight	•	•	•	•	•	•	•	•
Head Circumference	•	•	•	•	•	•	•	•
Blood Pressure								
SENSORY SCREENING								
Vision	S	S	S	S	S	S	S	S
Hearing	S	S	S	S	S	S	S	S
DEVELOP-MENTAL/ BEHAVIORAL ASSESSMENT[2]	•	•	•	•	•	•	•	•
PHYSICAL EXAMINATION[3]	•	•	•	•	•	•	•	•

1. *For newborns discharged in less than 48 hours after delivery*

2. *By history and appropriate physical examination: if suspicious, by specific objective development testing*

3. *At each visit, a complete physical examination is essential, with infant totally unclothed, older child undressed and suitably draped*

Key: • *to be performed; S = subjective, by history; O = objective, by a standard testing method*

RECOMMENDATIONS FOR PREVENTIVE PEDIATRIC CARE

Early Childhood AGE	15 mo	18 mo	24 mo	3 y	4y
HISTORY **Initial/Interval**	•	•	•	•	•
MEASUREMENTS **Height and Weight**	•	•	•	•	•
Head Circumference					
Blood Pressure	•	•	•	•	•
SENSORY SCREENING **Vision**	S	S	S	O	O
Hearing	S	S	S	O	O
DEVELOPMENTAL/ **BEHAVIORAL ASSESSMENT**[2]	•	•	•	•	•
PHYSICAL EXAMINATION[3]	•	•	•	•	•

Middle Childhood AGE	5 y	6 y	8 y	10 y
HISTORY **Initial/Interval**	•	•	•	•
MEASUREMENTS **Height and Weight**	•	•	•	•
Head Circumference				
Blood Pressure	•	•	•	•
SENSORY SCREENING **Vision**	O	S	S	O
Hearing	O	S	S	O
DEVELOPMENTAL/ **BEHAVIORAL ASSESSMENT**[2]	•	•	•	•
PHYSICAL EXAMINATION[3]	•	•	•	•

(continued)

Adolescence AGE	11 y	12 y	13 y	14 y	15 y
HISTORY Initial/Interval	•	•	•	•	•
MEASUREMENTS Height and Weight	•	•	•	•	•
Head Circumference					
Blood Pressure	•	•	•	•	•
SENSORY SCREENING Vision	S	O	S	S	O
Hearing	S	O	S	S	O
DEVELOPMENTAL/ BEHAVIORAL ASSESSMENT[2]	•	•	•	•	•
PHYSICAL EXAMINATION[3]	•	•	•	•	•

Adolescence AGE	16 y	17 y	18 y	19 y	20 y+
HISTORY Initial/Interval	•	•	•	•	•
MEASUREMENTS Height and Weight	•	•	•	•	•
Head Circumference					
Blood Pressure	•	•	•	•	•
SENSORY SCREENING Vision	S	S	O	S	S
Hearing	S	S	O	S	S
DEVELOPMENTAL/ BEHAVIORAL ASSESSMENT[2]	•	•	•	•	•
PHYSICAL EXAMINATION[3]	•	•	•	•	•

Adapted from Recommendations For Preventive Pediatric Health Care promulgated by the American Academy of Pediatrics Committee on Practice and Ambulatory Medicine. Pediatrics 96:373, 1995. Additional recommendations made by the Committee regarding screening for metabolic disorders, tuberculosis, anemia and urinary tract diseases, administration of immunizations, provision of anticipatory guidance, and initial dental referral are not included in the above summation.

AIDS TO
INTERPRETATION

HEIGHT AND WEIGHT TABLES FOR ADULTS AGE 25 AND OVER

Height (without shoes)	Weight in Pounds (without clothing)		
	Small Frame	*Medium Frame*	*Large Frame*
Men			
5'1"	105–113	111–122	119–134
5'2"	108–116	114–126	122–137
5'3"	111–119	117–129	125–141
5'4"	114–122	120–132	128–145
5'5"	117–126	123–136	131–149
5'6"	121–130	127–140	135–154
5'7"	125–134	131–145	140–159
5'8"	129–138	135–149	144–163
5'9"	133–143	139–153	148–167
5'10"	137–147	143–158	152–172
5'11"	141–151	147–163	157–177
6'0"	145–155	151–168	161–182
6'1"	149–160	155–173	168–187
6'2"	153–164	160–178	171–192
6'3"	157–168	165–183	175–197
Women			
4'9"	90–97	94–106	102–118
4'10"	92–100	97–109	106–121
4'11"	95–103	100–112	108–124
5'0"	98–106	103–116	111–127
5'1"	101–109	106–118	114–130
5'2"	104–112	109–122	117–134
5'3"	107–115	112–126	121–138
5'4"	110–119	116–131	125–142
5'5"	114–123	120–136	129–146
5'6"	118–127	124–139	133–150

(*continued*)

HEIGHT AND WEIGHT TABLES FOR ADULTS AGE 25 AND OVER
(Continued)

Height (without shoes)	Weight in Pounds (without clothing)		
	Small Frame	*Medium Frame*	*Large Frame*
Women			
5'7"	122–131	128–143	137–154
5'8"	126–136	132–147	141–159
5'9"	130–140	136–151	145–164
5'10"	134–144	140–155	149–169

From Clinician's Handbook of Preventive Services. Washington, DC: U.S. Department of Health and Human Services, 1994:142–143.

CLASSIFICATION OF A NEWBORN INFANT'S LEVEL OF MATURITY

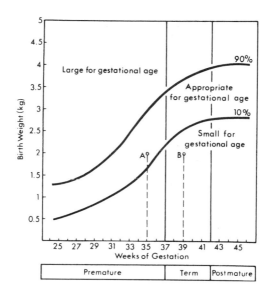

Weight Small for Gestational Age (SGA) = Birth weight <10th percentile on the intrauterine growth curve

Weight Appropriate for Gestational Age (AGA) = Birth weight within the 10th and 90th percentiles on the intrauterine growth curve

Weight Large for Gestational Age (LGA) = Birth weight >90th percentile on the intrauterine growth curve

Level of intrauterine growth based on birth weight and gestational age of liveborn, single, white infants. Point A represents a premature infant, while point B indicates an infant of similar birth weight who is mature but small for gestational age; the growth curves are representative of the 10th and 90th percentiles for all of the newborns in the sampling.

Classification of the low-birth-weight infant. In Klaus MH, Fanaroff AA: Care of the High-Rise Neonate, 3rd ed. Philadelphia, WB Saunders, 1986

HEIGHT AND WEIGHT GRIDS FOR GIRLS: BIRTH TO 36 MONTHS

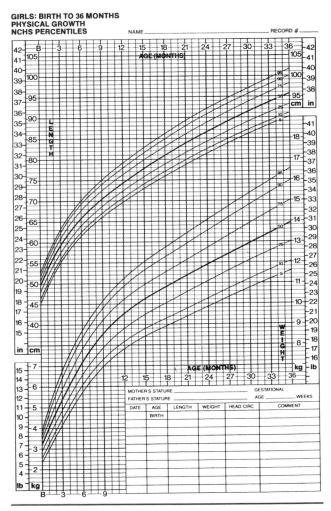

GIRLS: BIRTH TO 36 MONTHS
PHYSICAL GROWTH
NCHS PERCENTILES

(Adapted from Hamill PVV, Drizd TA, Johnson CL, Reed RB, Roche AF, Moore AM: Physical growth: National Center for Health Statistics percentiles. Am J Clin Nutr 32:607–629, 1979. Data from the National Center for Health Statistics [NCHS], Hyattsville, MD. Figures provided through the courtesy of Ross Laboratories, Columbus, OH)

HEIGHT AND WEIGHT GRIDS FOR GIRLS: 2 TO 18 YEARS

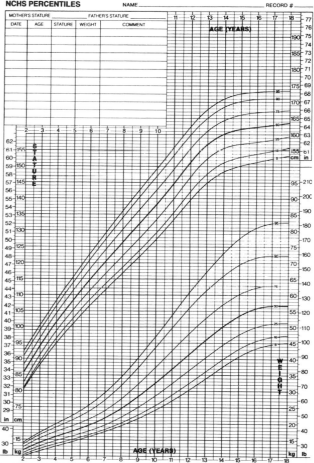

(Adapted from Hamill PVV, Drizd TA, Johnson CL, Reed RB, Roche AF, Moore AM: Physical growth: National Center for Health Statistics percentiles. Am J Clin Nutr 32:607–629, 1979. Data from the National Center for Health Statistics [NCHS], Hyattsville, MD. Figures provided through the courtesy of Ross Laboratories, Columbus, OH)

HEIGHT AND WEIGHT GRIDS FOR BOYS: BIRTH TO 36 MONTHS

BOYS: BIRTH TO 36 MONTHS
PHYSICAL GROWTH
NCHS PERCENTILES

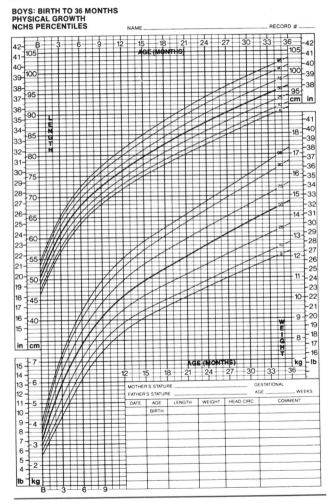

(Adapted from Hamill PVV, Drizd TA, Johnson CL, Reed RB, Roche AF, Moore AM: Physical growth: National Center for Health Statistics percentiles. Am J Clin Nutr 32:607–629, 1979. Data from the National Center for Health Statistics [NCHS], Hyattsville, MD. Figures provided through the courtesy of Ross Laboratories, Columbus, OH)

HEIGHT AND WEIGHT GRIDS FOR BOYS: 2 TO 18 YEARS

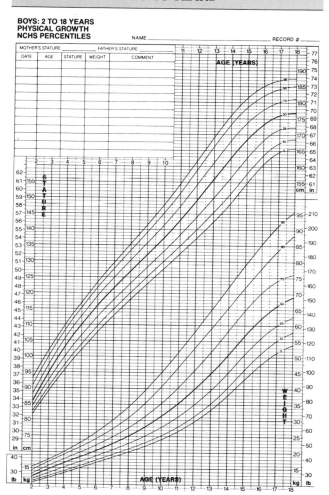

**BOYS: 2 TO 18 YEARS
PHYSICAL GROWTH
NCHS PERCENTILES**

(Adapted from Hamill PVV, Drizd TA, Johnson CL, Reed RB, Roche AF, Moore AM: Physical growth: National Center for Health Statistics percentiles. Am J Clin Nutr 32:607–629, 1979. Data from the National Center for Health Statistics [NCHS], Hyattsville, MD. Figures provided through the courtesy of Ross Laboratories, Columbus, OH)

BOYS: BIRTH TO 18 YEARS HEAD CIRCUMFERENCE GROWTH

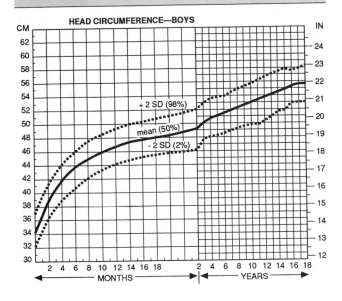

(Adapted from Nellhaus G: Composite international and interracial graphs. Pediatrics 41:106, 1968)

GIRLS: BIRTH TO 18 YEARS HEAD CIRCUMFERENCE GROWTH

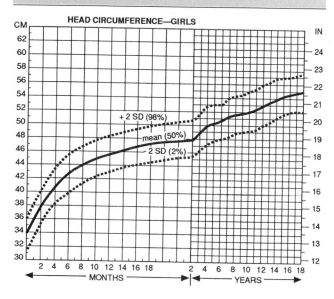

(Adapted from Nellhaus G: Composite international and interracial graphs. Pediatrics 41:106, 1968)

LEVELS OF CONSCIOUSNESS

Alertness
Awake, aware of self and environment. When spoken to in a normal voice, patient looks at you and responds fully and appropriately to stimuli.

Lethargy
When spoken to in a loud voice, patient appears drowsy but opens eyes and looks at you, responds to questions, then falls asleep.

Obtundation
When shaken gently, patient opens eyes and looks at you but responds slowly and is somewhat confused. Alertness and interest in environment decreased.

Stupor
Patient arouses from sleep only after painful stimuli. Verbal responses slow or absent. Lapses into unresponsiveness when stimulus stops. Minimal awareness of self or environment.

Coma
Despite repeated painful stimuli, patient remains unarousable with eyes closed. No evident response to inner need or external stimuli.

DISORDERS OF SPEECH

Aphonia/Dysphonia	A loss (aphonia) or impairment (dysphonia) of voice due to disease of larynx or its nerve supply. Volume, quality, and pitch of voice affected, as in hoarseness, whisper
Dysarthria	Defective muscular control of lips, tongue, palate, or pharynx, causing nasal, slurred, or indistinct speech. Symbolic aspect of language remains intact. Due to motor lesions in central or peripheral nervous system, parkinsonism, or cerebellar disease
Aphasia	A disorder in producing or understanding language, often due to lesions in the dominant cerebral hemisphere. Two common types:
	Wernicke's—Fluent, often rapid, voluble, effortless. Inflection and articulation good, but sentences lack meaning and words are malformed or invented.
	Broca's—Nonfluent, slow, effortful, with few words. Inflection and articulation impaired, but words meaningful with nouns, transitive verbs, important adjectives

DELIRIUM AND DEMENTIA

	Delirium	Dementia
Timing	Acute onset, fluctuating course, lasts hours/weeks	Insidious onset, slowly progressive, lasts months, years
Sleep pattern	Sleep/wake cycle disrupted	Sleep fragmented
Medical illness or drug toxicity	One or both present	Often absent, especially in Alzheimer's disease
Level of consciousness	Disturbed. Decreased awareness, attention	Usually normal until late in course
Activity	Often abnormally decreased or increased	Normal to slow, may be inappropriate
Speech	May be slow, hesitant, fast, incoherent	May be aphasic, show difficulty in finding words
Mood	Labile, may be irritable, fearful, depressed	Often flat, depressed
Thought processes	Disorganized, may be incoherent	Impoverished, with little information
Thought content	Delusions common, often transient	Delusions may occur.
Perceptions	Illusions, hallucinations	Hallucinations may occur.

(continued)

DELIRIUM AND DEMENTIA
(*Continued*)

	Delirium	Dementia
Orientation	Usually disoriented, especially for time. A known place may seem unfamiliar.	Fairly well maintained, but impaired late in course of illness
Attention	Fluctuates. Person easily distracted, unable to concentrate	Usually not affected until late in illness
Causes include:	Delirium tremens Uremia Acute liver failure Drug toxicity Hypoxia Hypoglycemia	*Reversible:* Vitamin B_{12} deficiency Thyroid disorders *Irreversible:* Alzheimer's disease Vascular dementia Head trauma

COLOR CHANGES IN THE SKIN

Color/Mechanism	Selected Causes
Brown: Increased melanin (greater than a person's genetic norm)	Sun exposure Pregnancy (melasma) Addison's disease
Blue (cyanosis): Increased deoxyhemoglobin due to hypoxia:	
• Peripheral	Anxiety or cold environment
• Central (arterial)	Heart or lung disease
Abnormal hemoglobin	Methemoglobinemia, sulfhemoglobinemia
Red: Increased visibility of oxyhemoglobin due to:	
Dilated superficial blood vessels or increased blood flow in skin	Fever, blushing, alcohol intake, local inflammation
Decreased use of oxygen in skin	Cold exposure (e.g., cold ears)
Yellow:	
Increased bilirubin of jaundice (sclera looks yellow)	Liver disease, hemolysis of red blood cells
Carotenemia (sclera does not look yellow)	Increased carotene intake from yellow fruits and vegetables
Pale: Decreased melanin	Albinism, vitiligo, tinea versicolor
Decreased visibility of oxyhemoglobin due to:	
• Decreased blood flow to skin	Syncope or shock
• Decreased amount of oxyhemoglobin	Anemia
Edema (may mask skin pigments)	Nephrotic syndrome

TYPES OF SKIN LESIONS

Primary Lesions

Circumscribed, flat, nonpalpable changes in color:

MACULE. Small spot. Examples: freckle, petechia

PATCH. Larger macule. Example: vitiligo

Palpable, elevated, solid masses:

PAPULE. Up to 0.5 cm. Example: the papule of acne.

PLAQUE. An elevated flat surface larger than 0.5 cm. Example: xanthelasma of the eyelids

NODULE. Larger than 0.5 cm; often deeper and firmer than a papule. Example: epidermoid cyst

TUMOR. Large nodule. Example: a large neurofibroma

WHEAL. A relatively transient, superficial area of local skin edema. Example: mosquito bite

Circumscribed superficial elevations of the skin formed by free fluid in a cavity between the skin layers:

VESICLE. Up to 0.5 cm; filled with serous fluid. Example: poison ivy

BULLA. Greater than 0.5 cm; filled with serous fluid. Example: 2nd-degree burn

PUSTULE. Filled with pus. Example: acne

(continued)

TYPES OF SKIN LESIONS
(*Continued*)

Secondary Lesions

Loss of skin surface:

EROSION. Loss of superficial epidermis, leaving a moist area that does not bleed. Example: skin surface after a ruptured vesicle

ULCER. A deeper loss of surface that may bleed and scar. Examples: syphilitic chancre, ulcer of venous insufficiency

FISSURE. A linear crack. Example: athlete's foot

Material on the skin surface:

CRUST. The dried residue of serum, pus, or blood. Example: a scab

SCALE. A thin flake of exfoliated epidermis. Examples: dry skin, dandruff

CHARACTERISTICS OF MOLES

Normal

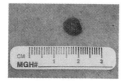

Diameter smaller than 6 millimeters
Symmetrical; regular borders, even in color

Malignant melanoma

(ABCDE)

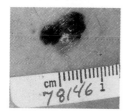

Asymmetrical

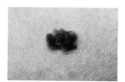

Borders irregular

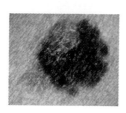

Color varied
Diameter more than 6 mm
Elevation

(Courtesy of American Cancer Society; American Academy of Dermatology)

FINGERNAILS

Clubbing

Dorsal phalanx rounded and bulbous; convexity of nail plate increased. Angle between plate and proximal nail fold increased to 180° or more. Proximal nail folds feel spongy. Many causes, including chronic hypoxia and lung cancer

Paronychia

Inflammation of proximal and lateral nail folds, acute or chronic. Folds red, swollen, may be tender.

Onycholysis

Painless separation of nail plate from nail bed, starting distally. Many causes.

Terry's nails

Whitish with a distal band of reddish brown. Seen in aging and some chronic diseases.

(*continued*)

FINGERNAILS

Leukonychia

White spots caused by trauma. They grow out with nail(s).

Transverse white lines

Curved white lines similar to curve of lunula. They follow an illness and grow out with nails.

Beau's lines

Transverse depressions in nails that follow an illness and grow out with nails.

Pitting

Small pits in nail plates. May accompany psoriasis and some other conditions.

VISUAL FIELD DEFECTS

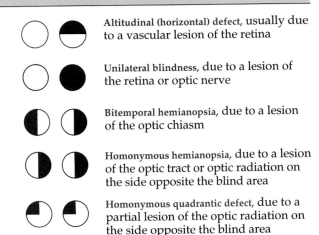

Altitudinal (horizontal) defect, usually due to a vascular lesion of the retina

Unilateral blindness, due to a lesion of the retina or optic nerve

Bitemporal hemianopsia, due to a lesion of the optic chiasm

Homonymous hemianopsia, due to a lesion of the optic tract or optic radiation on the side opposite the blind area

Homonymous quadrantic defect, due to a partial lesion of the optic radiation on the side opposite the blind area

LEFT   RIGHT

(from patient's viewpoint)

PHYSICAL FINDINGS IN AND AROUND THE EYE

Herniated fat. A common cause of swelling in the lower lid and the inner third of the upper lid; associated with aging

Periorbital edema. Swelling of the eyelids from excessive fluid; many causes, including cellulitis, nephrotic syndrome

Ptosis. A drooping upper eyelid that narrows the palpebral fissure; due to a muscle or nerve disorder

Enlarged palpebral fissure. Seen in retraction of the eyelids, exophthalmos, both signs of hyperthyroidism

Ectropion. Outward turning of the margin of the lower lid, exposing the palpebral conjunctiva

Entropion. Inward turning of the lid margin, causing irritation of the cornea or conjunctiva

Pingueculae. Harmless yellowish nodules in the bulbar conjunctiva on either side of the iris; associated with aging

Xanthelasma. Yellowish plaques in the eyelids that may be due to a lipid disorder

(*continued*)

PHYSICAL FINDINGS IN AND AROUND THE EYE (*Continued*)

Basal cell epithelioma. A common skin cancer

Chalazion. A beady nodule in either eyelid due to a chronically inflamed meibomian gland

Sty. A pimplelike infection around a hair follicle near the lid margin

Dacryocystitis. An inflammation of the lacrimal sac, acute or chronic, that may obstruct tear drainage

Corneal arcus. A grayish white arc or ring often associated with aging

Pterygium. A thickening of the bulbar conjunctiva that may grow across the cornea

RED EYES

	Pain	Vision	Ocular Discharge	Pupil	Cornea
Conjunctivitis	Mild or no discomfort	Only temporary blurring from discharge	Present	Normal	Clear
Ciliary injection					
OF CORNEAL ORIGIN	Present, superficial	Usually decreased	Present	Normal, unless iritis ensues	Varies with cause
ACUTE IRITIS	Present, aching, deep	Decreased	Absent	Small	Clear or slightly clouded
ACUTE GLAUCOMA	Severe, aching, deep	Decreased	Absent	Dilated, fixed	Steamy, cloudy
Subconjunctival hemorrhage	Absent	Normal	Absent	Normal	Clear

PUPILLARY ABNORMALITIES

Blind eye. Neither a direct nor a consensual response to light occurs when this blind left eye is stimulated. Normal responses occur when the normal right eye is so stimulated.

Marcus Gunn (deafferented) pupil. Diminished direct and consensual responses occur when an eye impaired by an optic nerve disorder is stimulated by light. Testing this normal right eye causes normal responses. When the light is swung back to the impaired left eye, the pupils dilate.

Horner's Syndrome. A small pupil due to interruption of its sympathetic nerve supply. Ptosis is associated. Pupillary reactions are normal.

Oculomotor nerve paralysis. A large pupil, often associated with ptosis of the lid and lateral deviation of the eye. Pupillary reactions absent in that eye

Tonic pupil. A large pupil with decreased or absent reaction to light and a slow response to near effort

Argyll Robertson pupils. Small, irregular pupils that react to near effort but not to light

Dilated fixed pupils. Associated with drug effects or severe brain damage

Small fixed pupils. Associated with miotic eye drops, drugs, or brain damage at the level of the pons

ABNORMALITIES OF THE OPTIC DISC

	Process	Appearance
Normal 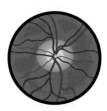	Tiny disc vessels give normal color to the disc.	Color yellowish orange to creamy pink Disc vessels tiny Disc margins sharp (except perhaps nasally)
Optic Atrophy 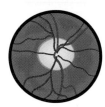	Death of optic nerve fibers leads to loss of the tiny disc vessels.	Color white Disc vessels absent
Papilledema 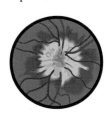	Venous stasis leads to engorge-ment and swelling.	Color pink, hyperemic Disc vessels more visible, more numerous, curve over the borders of the disc Disc swollen with margins blurred

(*continued*)

ABNORMALITIES OF THE OPTIC DISC
(*Continued*)

	Process	Appearance
Glaucomatous cupping 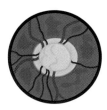	Increased pressure within the eye leads to increased cupping (backward depression of the disc) and atrophy.	The base of the enlarged cup is pale.

RETINAL LESIONS

Preretinal hemorrhage

Anterior to the retina, develops when blood escapes into potential space between retina and vitreous

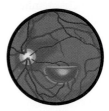

Superficial retinal hemorrhages

Small linear, flame-shaped red streaks in the fundus. Linear streaking at edge is distinguishing characteristic.

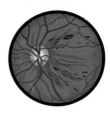

Deep retinal hemorrhages

Small rounded, slightly irregular red spots, occurring in a deeper layer of retina

(*continued*)

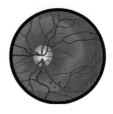

RETINAL LESIONS
(*Continued*)

Microaneurysms

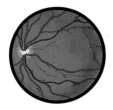

Tiny red spots, seen commonly in and around macula, which are minute dilations of very small retinal vessels

Hypertensive retinopathy

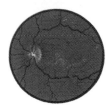

Nasal border of the optic disk is blurred. "Silver wiring" of arteries above and below disk from increased light reflexes. AV nicking with venous tapering and AV crossing one disk diameter above the disk. Punctate hard exudates and scattered deep hemorrhages present.

Diabetic retinopathy

NONPROLIFERATIVE RETINOPATHY, MODERATELY SEVERE.

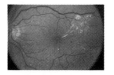

Note tiny red dots or microaneurysms. Note also the ring of hard exudates (white spots) located superotemporally. Retinal thickening or edema in the area of the hard exudates can impair visual acuity if it extends into the center of the macula (detection requires specialized stereoscopic examination).

(*continued*)

RETINAL LESIONS

NONPROLIFERATIVE RETINOPATHY, SEVERE

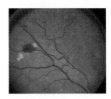

In the superior temporal quadrant, note the large retinal hemorrhage between two cotton-wool patches, beading of the retinal vein (just above them), and tiny tortuous retinal vessels above the superior temporal artery (termed *intraretinal microvascular abnormalities*).

PROLIFERATIVE RETINOPATHY, WITH NEOVASCULARIZATION

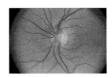

Note new preretinal vessels arising on the disc and extending across the disc margins. Visual acuity is currently normal, but risk of severe visual loss is high. (This risk can be reduced more than 50% with photocoagulation.)

PROLIFERATIVE RETINOPATHY, ADVANCED

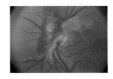

Same eye as above, but 2 years later and without treatment. Neovascularization has increased, now with fibrous proliferations, distortion of the macula, and reduced visual acuity.

(Source: Early Treatment Diabetic Retinopathy Study Research Group. Courtesy of M. F. Davis, MD, University of Wisconsin, Madison.)

LUMPS ON OR NEAR THE EAR

Chondrodermatitis helicis
Painful, tender, chronic papule on helix or possibly antihelix. May ulcerate and crust.

Squamous cell carcinoma
Growing papule that may ulcerate and crust, most often on helix. Light skin and sun exposure predispose.

Epidermoid cyst
A smooth, rounded cyst, often with a dark dot (punctum) that marks the opening of a sebaceous gland. May become inflamed. Often behind the ear.

Basal cell carcinoma
A slow-growing nodule with a lustrous surface and telangiectatic vessels. May ulcerate.

Lumps with chronic arthritis
Consider a rheumatoid nodule that accompanies rheumatoid arthritis or a tophus of chronic tophaceous gout. The latter discharges white chalky crystals of uric acid.

Keloid
A nodular hypertrophic mass of scar tissue that follows injury such as piercing the ears. Darker-skinned people more susceptible.

Enlarged lymph nodes
The preauricular and postauricular nodes, when enlarged, may cause lumps beneath the skin in front of and behind the ear respectively.

ABNORMAL EARDRUMS

Serous effusion

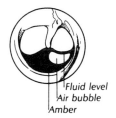

Fluid level
Air bubble
Amber

Amber fluid behind the eardrum, with or without air bubbles

Associated with viral upper respiratory infections or sudden changes in atmospheric pressure (diving, flying)

Acute otitis media

Red, bulging drum, loss of landmarks

Associated with bacterial infection

Tympanosclerosis

A chalky white patch

Scar of an old otitis media; of little or no clinical consequence

Perforation

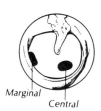

Marginal
Central

Hole in the eardrum that may be central or marginal

Usually the result of otitis media or trauma

PATTERNS OF HEARING LOSS

	Conductive Loss	Sensorineural Loss
Impaired under-standing of words	Minor	Often troublesome
Effect of noisy environment	May help	Increases the hearing difficulty
Usual age of onset	Childhood, young adulthood	Middle and old age
Ear canal and drum	Often a visible abnormality	The problem not visible
Weber's test (in unilateral hearing loss)	Lateralizes to the impaired ear	Lateralizes to the good ear
Rinne test	BC > AC or BC = AC	AC > BC
Causes include:	Plugged ear canal Otitis media Immobile or perforated drum Otosclerosis	Sustained loud noise, drugs, inner ear infections, trauma, hereditary dis-order, aging

ABNORMALITIES OF THE LIPS

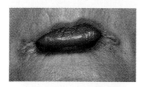

Angular cheilitis. Softening and cracking of the angles of the mouth

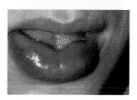

Angioedema. Diffuse, tense, subcutaneous swelling, usually allergic in cause

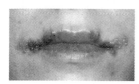

Herpes simplex (cold sore, fever blister). Painful vesicles, followed by crusting

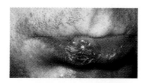

Syphilitic chancre. A firm lesion that ulcerates and may crust

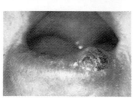

Carcinoma of the lip. A thickened plaque or irregular nodule that may ulcerate or crust. Malignant.

(continued)

ABNORMALITIES OF THE LIPS
(*Continued*)

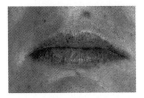

Hereditary hemorrhagic telangiectasia. Red spots, significant because of associated bleeding from nose and GI tract

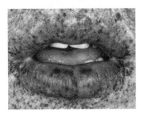

Peutz-Jeghers syndrome. Brown spots of the lips and buccal mucosa, significant because of their association with intestinal polyposis

ABNORMALITIES OF THE GUMS AND TEETH

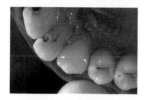

Dental caries. Tooth decay. Clinically invisible in its early stages, it may produce chalky white spots that later discolor to brown or black, soften and cavitate.

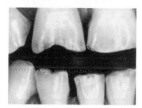

Abrasion of teeth. Irregularities in the biting edges due to recurrent trauma

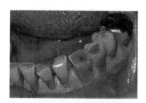

Attrition of teeth. Wear of the teeth. The exposed dentin is often yellow or brown.

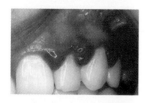

Marginal gingivitis. Red, swollen gum margins with blunted interdental papilla

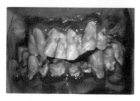

Periodontitis. A progression of gingivitis to deeper tissues, with resulting recession of the gums and looseness or loss of teeth

(continued)

ABNORMALITIES OF THE GUMS AND TEETH
(*Continued*)

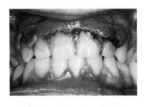

Acute necrotizing ulcerative gingivitis. Red, painful gums with marginal ulceration and a grayish pseudomembrane. Foul breath, fever, lymphadenopathy

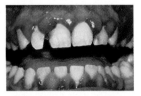

Gingival enlargement. Enlarged gums that partially cover the teeth with heaped-up tissue

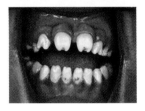

Hutchinson's teeth. A sign of congenital syphilis; most often involving the upper central incisors. These teeth are small, notched, tapered, and widely spaced.

TONGUES

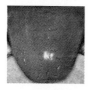

Smooth tongue. Due to loss of papillae, caused by vitamin B or iron deficiency, or possibly anticancer drugs

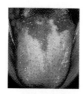

Hairy tongue. Due to elongated papillae that may look yellowish, brown, or black. Harmless

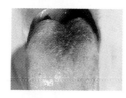

Geographic tongue. Scattered areas in which the papillae are lost, giving a map-like appearance. Harmless

Fissured tongue. Fissues may appear with aging. Harmless

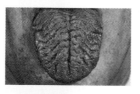

Varicose veins (caviar lesions). Dark round spots in the undersurface of the tongue, associated with aging

(*continued*)

TONGUES
(*Continued*)

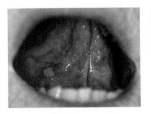

Apthous ulcer (canker sore). Painful small, whitish ulcer with a red halo. Heals in 7 to 10 days

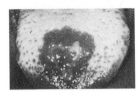

Candida infection. May show a thick, white coat, which, when scraped off, leaves a raw red surface. Tongue may also be red. Antibiotics, corticosteroids, AIDS may predispose

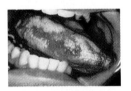

Hairy leukoplakia. White raised, feathery areas, usually on sides of tongue

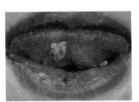

Mucous patch of syphilis. Slightly raised, oval lesion, covered by a grayish membrane

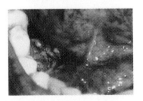

Carcinoma of the tongue or floor of the mouth. A malignancy that should be considered in any nodule or nonhealing ulcer at the base or edges of the mouth.

ABNORMALITIES OF THE PHARYNX

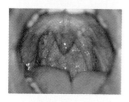

Pharyngitis, mild to moderate. Note redness and vascularity of the pillars and uvula.

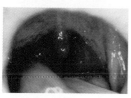

Pharyngitis, diffuse. Note redness is diffuse and intense. Cause may be viral or, if patient has fever, bacterial. If patient has no fever, exudate, or cervical lymphadenopathy, viral infection is more likely.

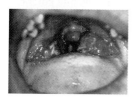

Exudative pharyngitis. A sore red throat with patches of white exudate on the tonsils is associated with streptococcal pharyngitis and some viral illnesses, including infectious mononucleosis. In diptheria, unlike streptococcal infections, the exudate may spread as a gray membrane over the soft palate and uvula.

Peritonsillar abscess. A unilateral red bulge in the pharynx that may displace the uvula toward the opposite side.

Unilateral palatal weakness with deviation of the uvula. Seen in unilateral paralysis of the vagal nerve, often from stroke. With "ah," the soft palate fails to rise on the affected side and the uvula deviates to the opposite side.

ABNORMALITIES OF THE HARD PALATE

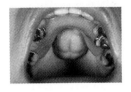

Torus palatinus. A midline bony outgrowth in the hard palate. Size and lobulation vary from person to person. Harmless

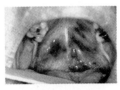

Kaposi's sarcoma. A mass in the palate, especially when not midline, may be a tumor such as Kaposi's sarcoma in AIDS. The classic purple-red color may not be present.

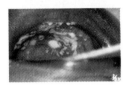

Candida infection. White patches that can be scraped off suggest this diagnosis.

ABNORMALITIES OF THE THYROID GLAND

 Diffuse Enlargement. May be due to Graves' disease, Hashimoto's thyroiditis, endemic goiter (iodine deficiency), or sporadic goiter

 Multinodular Goiter. An enlargement with two or more identifiable nodules, usually metabolic in cause.

 Single nodule. May be due to a cyst, a benign tumor, or cancer of the thyroid, or may be one palpable nodule in a clinically unrecognized multinodular goiter.

ABNORMALITIES OF THYROID FUNCTION

Hyperthyroidism	Hypothyroidism
Nervousness	Fatigue
Weight loss	Weight gain
Sweating, heat intolerance; skin warm, smooth, moist	Dry skin, cold intolerance, hair loss, nonpitting edema
Frequent stools	Constipation
Tremor, proximal weakness	Weakness; poor memory, hearing
Tachycardia, atrial fibrillation	Bradycardia; hypothermia (late)
In Graves' disease, stare, lid lag, exophthalmos	Periorbital edema

RATE AND RHYTHM OF BREATHING

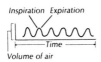

Normal. In adults, 14 to 20 per minute; in infants, up to 40 per minute

‖‖‖‖‖‖‖‖‖‖‖‖

Rapid Shallow Breathing (Tachypnea). Many causes, including restrictive lung disease and pleural pain

Rapid Deep Breathing (Hyperpnea, hyperventilation). Many causes, including exercise, anxiety, metabolic acidosis, brainstem injury. *Kussmaul breathing,* due to metabolic acidosis, is deep but rate may be fast, slow, or normal.

Slow Breathing. May be due to diabetic coma, drug-induced respiratory depression, increased intracranial pressure

Hyperpnea   Apnea

Cheyne-Stokes Breathing. Rhythmically alternating periods of hyperpnea and apnea. In infants and the aged, may be normal during sleep; also accompanies brain damage, heart failure, uremia, and respiratory depression

Ataxic (Biot's) Breathing. Unpredictable irregularity of depth and rate. Causes include brain damage and respiratory depression

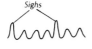

Sighing Breathing. Breathing punctuated by frequent sighs. When associated with other symptoms, it suggests the hyperventilation syndrome. Occasional sighs are normal.

DEFORMITIES OF THE THORAX

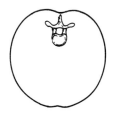

Barrel Chest. An anteroposterior diameter increased from the adult norm so that the chest (in cross-section) becomes rounded. May accompany aging and chronic obstructive pulmonary disease. (The chest of a normal infant also has this shape).

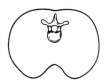

Funnel Chest (Pectis Excavatum). Posterior displacement of the lower sternum. Compression of the heart or great vessels may cause murmurs.

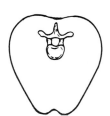

Pigeon Chest (Pectus Carinatum). Anterior displacement of the sternum. The costal cartilages adjacent to the sternum are relatively depressed.

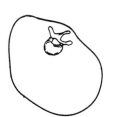

Thoracic Kyphoscoliosis. A structural spinal curvature that may be associated with distortion and asymmetry of the chest.

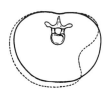

Flail Chest. Abnormal respiratory movements associated with multiple rib fractures. The injured area moves inward in inspiration, outward in expiration.

LUNG LOBES

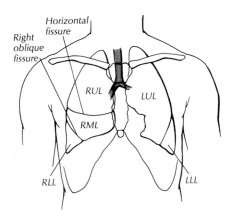

ANTERIOR

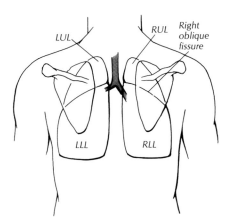

POSTERIOR

PERCUSSION NOTES

	Relative Intensity, Pitch, and Duration	Examples
Flatness	Soft/high/short	Large pleural effusion
Dullness	Medium/medium/medium	Lobar pneumonia
Resonance	Loud/low/long	Normal lung, simple chronic bronchitis
Hyperresonance	Louder, lower, longer	Emphysema, pneumothorax
Tympany	Loud/high*/*	Large pneumothorax

*Distinguished mainly by musical timbre

BREATH SOUNDS

	Duration	Intensity and Pitch of Expiratory Sound	Example Locations
Vesicular	Insp > exp	Soft/low	Most of the lungs
Bronchovesicular	Insp = exp	Medium/medium	1st and 2nd interspaces, interscapular area
Bronchial	Exp > insp	Loud/high	Over the manubrium; lobar pneumonia
Tracheal	Insp = exp	Very loud/high	Over the trachea

In the figures above, duration is indicated by the length of the line, intensity by the width of the line, and pitch by the slope of the line.

TRANSMITTED VOICE SOUNDS

Through Normally Air-Filled Lung	Through Airless Lung*
Spoken words muffled and indistinct	Spoken words louder, clearer (*bronchophony*)
Spoken "ee" heard as "ee"	Spoken "ee" heard as "ay" (*egophony*)
Whispered words faint and indistinct, if heard at all	Whispered words louder, clearer (*whispered pectoriloquy*)
Usually accompanied by vesicular breath sounds and normal tactile fremitus	Usually accompanied by bronchial or bronchovesicular breath sounds and increased tactile fremitus

*As in lobar pneumonia and toward the top of a large pleural effusion

ADVENTITIOUS LUNG SOUNDS

Discontinuous sounds (crackles)

Intermittent, nonmusical, short sounds, like dots in time

- *Fine crackles* (· · · ·)—soft, high in pitch, very brief

- *Coarse crackles* (••••)—somewhat louder, lower in pitch, not quite so brief

CRACKLES CLASSIFIED BY TIMING

- *Late inspiratory crackles.* Must continue into late inspiration. Usually fine, profuse, and heard in dependent portions of the lungs. Causes include interstitial lung disease and early congestive heart failure.

- *Early inspiratory crackles.* Do not continue into late inspiration. Often coarse. Causes include chronic bronchitis and asthma.

Continuous sounds

Musical and notably longer than crackles, like dashes in time, but not necessarily truly continuous. May be generalized (as in asthma or chronic obstructive lung disease) or persistent and local (as from a tumor or foreign body that is obstructing a bronchus). Clearing by cough or deep breathing suggests secretions as the cause.

- *Wheezes* (ᴧᴧᴧᴧᴧ)—relatively high in pitch (around 400 Hz or more), with a hissing or shrill quality

- *Rhonchi* (ᴧᴧᴧᴧ)—relatively low in pitch (around 200 Hz or less), with a snoring quality

Stridor

A high-pitched wheeze heard only or chiefly in inspiration and often louder in the neck than over the chest. Indicates partial airway obstruction in the neck

(continued)

ADVENTITIOUS LUNG SOUNDS

Pleural rub

A creaking, grating sound associated with respiratory movements. Originates in inflamed pleural surfaces

Mediastinal crunch

A series of precordial crackles synchronous with the heart beat, heard best in the left lateral position. Due to mediastinal emphysema (pneumomediastinum)

SIGNS IN SELECTED CHEST DISORDERS

	Trachea	Percussion Note
Chronic bronchitis	Midline	Resonant
Left heart failure (early)	Midline	Resonant
Consolidation*	Midline	Dull
Atelectasis (Lobar)	May be shifted toward	Dull
Pleural effusion (large)	May be shifted away	Dull
Pneumothorax	May be shifted away	Hyperresonant or tympanitic
Emphysema	Midline	Hyperresonant
Asthma	Midline	Normal to hyperresonant

*As in lobar pneumonia, pulmonary edema, or pulmonary hemorrhage

Breath Sounds	Transmitted Voice Sounds	Adventitious Sounds
Normal	Normal	None, or wheezes, rhonchi, crackles
Normal	Normal	Late inspiratory crackles in lower lungs; possible wheezes
Bronchial	Increased*	Late inspiratory crackles
Usually absent	Usually absent	None
Decreased to absent	Decreased to absent	Usually none, possible pleural rub
Decreased to absent	Decreased to absent	Possible pleural rub
Decreased to absent	Decreased	None unless bronchitis also
May be obscured by wheezes	Decreased	Wheezes, perhaps crackles

*With increased tactile fremitus, bronchophony, egophony, whispered pectoriloquy

COMMON BREAST NODULES

	Fibroadenoma	Gross Cyst	Cancer
Usual age	15–25 years (puberty and young adulthood) up to age 55	30–60 years	30–90 years
Number	Usually may be multiple	Single or multiple	Usually single; other nodules may coexist
Shape	Round, disclike, or lobular	Round	Irregular or stellate
Consistency	May be soft, usually firm	Soft to firm, usually elastic	Firm or hard
Delimitation	Well circumscribed	Well circumscribed	Not clearly delineated from surrounding tissues
Mobility	Very mobile	Mobile	May be fixed
Tenderness	Usually nontender	Often tender	Usually nontender
Retraction signs	Absent	Absent	May be present; overlying skin may have "peau d'orange" appearance

HEART RATES AND RHYTHMS

Regular rhythms

FAST (OVER 100)

Sinus tachycardia

Atrial or nodal (supraventricular) tachycardia

Atrial flutter with a regular ventricular response

Ventricular tachycardia

NORMAL (60–100)

Normal sinus rhythm

Second-degree AV block

Atrial flutter with a regular ventricular response

SLOW (< 50)

Sinus bradycardia

Second-degree AV block

Complete heart block

Irregular rhythms

RHYTHMICALLY OR SPORADICALLY IRREGULAR

Premature contractions (atrial, nodal, or ventricular)

Sinus arrhythmia

TOTALLY IRREGULAR

Atrial fibrillation

Atrial flutter with varying block

AVERAGE HEART RATE OF INFANTS AND CHILDREN AT REST

Age	Average Rate	Range (Two Standard Deviations)
Birth	140	90–190
1st 6 months	130	80–180
6–12 months	115	75–155
1–2 years	110	70–150
2–6 years	103	68–138
6–10 years	95	65–125
10–14 years	85	55–115

BLOOD PRESSURE IN ADULTS

Recommended size of the inflatable bag

- Width 40% of the arm circumference
- Length 80% of the arm circumference

Systolic pressure: The appearance point of Korotkoff sounds

Diastolic pressure: The disappearance point of Korotkoff sounds in adults, the muffle point in children

Methods of intensifying Korotkoff sounds

1. Raise patient's arm before and during inflation; then lower arm and take blood pressure.
2. Inflate cuff, ask patient to make a fist several times, and take blood pressure.

Blood Pressure Classification (Adults)*

Category	Systolic (mm Hg)	Diastolic (mm Hg)
Hypertension		
Stage 3 (severe)	≥180	≥110
Stage 2 (moderate)	160–179	100–109
Stage 1 (mild)	140–159	90–99
High Normal	130–139	85–89
Normal	<130	<85
Optimal	<120	<80

*When the systolic and diastolic levels indicate different categories, use the higher category. For example, 170/92 mm Hg is moderate hypertension and 170/120 mm Hg is severe hypertension.

In isolated systolic hypertension, *systolic pressure is 140 mm Hg or more and diastolic pressure is less than 90 mm Hg.*

Orthostatic (postural) hypotension: *A decrease of 20 mm Hg or more in systolic pressure, especially when accompanied by symptoms, after the patient changes from the supine to a sitting or standing position.*

BLOOD PRESSURE IN CHILDREN

Recommended size of the inflatable bag

- Width 90% of the upper arm or thigh circumference at its midpoint
- Length 80% to 100% or more of the upper arm or thigh circumference at its midpoint

Method

Same as for adults in children age 3 years and older

Use flush method for infants and younger children (see p. 114).

Classification of blood pressure levels in children

NORMAL: Systolic and diastolic BPs < 90th percentile for age and sex

HIGH NORMAL: Average systolic and diastolic BPs between the 90th and 95th percentiles for age and sex

HIGH (HYPERTENSION): Average systolic and/or diastolic BPs ≥95th percentile for age and sex

Blood Pressure Levels for the 90th and 95th Percentiles of Blood Pressure for Boys Aged 1 to 17 Years by Percentiles of Height

Boys Age, y	Blood Pressure Percentile*	Systolic Blood Pressure by Percentile of Height, mm Hg[†]						
		5%	10%	25%	50%	75%	90%	95%
1	90th	94	95	97	98	100	102	102
	95th	98	99	101	102	104	106	106
2	90th	98	99	100	102	104	105	106
	95th	101	102	104	106	108	109	110
3	90th	100	101	103	105	107	108	109
	95th	104	105	107	109	111	112	113
4	90th	102	103	105	107	109	110	111
	95th	106	107	109	111	113	114	115
5	90th	104	105	106	108	110	112	112
	95th	108	109	110	112	114	115	116

(*continued*)

BLOOD PRESSURE IN CHILDREN

Boys Age, y	Blood Pressure Percentile*	Systolic Blood Pressure by Percentile of Height, mm Hg†						
		5%	10%	25%	50%	75%	90%	95%
6	90th	105	106	108	110	111	113	114
	95th	109	110	112	114	115	117	117
7	90th	106	107	109	111	113	114	115
	95th	110	111	113	115	116	118	119
8	90th	107	108	110	112	114	115	116
	95th	111	112	114	116	118	119	120
9	90th	109	110	112	113	115	117	117
	95th	113	114	116	117	119	121	121
10	90th	110	112	113	115	117	118	119
	95th	114	115	117	119	121	122	123
11	90th	112	113	115	117	119	120	121
	95th	116	117	119	121	123	124	125
12	90th	115	116	117	119	121	123	123
	95th	119	120	121	123	125	126	127
13	90th	117	118	120	122	124	125	126
	95th	121	122	124	126	128	129	130
14	90th	120	121	123	125	126	128	128
	95th	124	125	127	128	130	132	132
15	90th	123	124	125	127	129	131	131
	95th	127	128	129	131	133	134	135
16	90th	125	126	128	130	132	133	134
	95th	129	130	132	134	136	137	138
17	90th	128	129	131	133	134	136	136
	95th	132	133	135	136	138	140	140

(*continued*)

BLOOD PRESSURE IN CHILDREN
(*Continued*)

Boys Age, y	Blood Pressure Percentile*	Diastolic Blood Pressure by Percentile of Height, mm Hg†						
		5%	10%	25%	50%	75%	90%	95%
1	90th	50	51	52	53	54	54	55
	95th	55	55	56	57	58	59	59
2	90th	55	55	56	57	58	59	59
	95th	59	59	60	61	62	63	63
3	90th	59	59	60	61	62	63	63
	95th	63	63	64	65	66	67	67
4	90th	62	62	63	64	65	66	66
	95th	66	67	67	68	69	70	71
5	90th	65	65	66	67	68	69	69
	95th	69	70	70	71	72	73	74
6	90th	67	68	69	70	70	71	72
	95th	72	72	73	74	75	76	76
7	90th	69	70	71	72	72	73	74
	95th	74	74	75	76	77	78	78
8	90th	71	71	72	73	74	75	75
	95th	75	76	76	77	78	79	80
9	90th	72	73	73	74	75	76	77
	95th	76	77	78	79	80	80	81
10	90th	73	74	74	75	76	77	78
	95th	77	78	79	80	80	81	82
11	90th	74	74	75	76	77	78	78
	95th	78	79	79	80	81	82	83
12	90th	75	75	76	77	78	78	79
	95th	79	79	80	81	82	83	83
13	90th	75	76	76	77	78	79	80
	95th	79	80	81	82	83	83	84

(*continued*)

BLOOD PRESSURE IN CHILDREN

Boys Age, y	Blood Pressure Percentile*	Diastolic Blood Pressure by Percentile of Height, mm Hg†						
		5%	10%	25%	50%	75%	90%	95%
14	90th	76	76	77	78	79	80	80
	95th	80	81	81	82	83	84	85
15	90th	77	77	78	79	80	81	81
	95th	81	82	83	83	84	85	86
16	90th	79	79	80	81	82	82	83
	95th	83	83	84	85	86	87	87
17	90th	81	81	82	83	84	85	85
	95th	85	85	86	87	88	89	89

Blood pressure percentile was determined by a single measurement.

†*Height percentile was determined by standard growth curves.*

Reproduced with permission from Update on the 1987 Task Force Report on High Blood Pressure in Children and Adolescents: A Working Group Report from the National High Blood Pressure Education Program. Pediatrics 98:649, 1996.

(continued)

BLOOD PRESSURE IN CHILDREN
(*Continued*)

Blood Pressure Levels for the 90th and 95th Percentiles of Blood
Pressure for Girls Aged 1 to 17 Years by Percentiles of Height

Girls Age, y	Blood Pressure Percentile*	Systolic Blood Pressure by Percentile of Height, mm Hg[†]						
		5%	10%	25%	50%	75%	90%	95%
1	90th	97	98	99	100	102	103	104
	95th	101	102	103	104	105	107	107
2	90th	99	99	100	102	103	104	105
	95th	102	103	104	105	107	108	109
3	90th	100	100	102	103	104	105	106
	95th	104	104	105	107	108	109	110
4	90th	101	102	103	104	106	107	108
	95th	105	106	107	108	109	111	111
5	90th	103	103	104	106	107	108	109
	95th	107	107	108	110	111	112	113
6	90th	104	105	106	107	109	110	111
	95th	108	109	110	111	112	114	114
7	90th	106	107	108	109	110	112	112
	95th	110	110	112	113	114	115	116
8	90th	108	109	110	111	112	113	114
	95th	112	112	113	115	116	117	118
9	90th	110	110	112	113	114	115	116
	95th	114	114	115	117	118	119	120
10	90th	112	112	114	115	116	117	118
	95th	116	116	117	119	120	121	122
11	90th	114	114	116	117	118	119	120
	95th	118	118	119	121	122	123	124
12	90th	116	116	118	119	120	121	122
	95th	120	120	121	123	124	125	126

(*continued*)

BLOOD PRESSURE IN CHILDREN

Girls Age, y	Blood Pressure Percentile*	Systolic Blood Pressure by Percentile of Height, mm Hg†						
		5%	10%	25%	50%	75%	90%	95%
13	90th	118	118	119	121	122	123	124
	95th	121	122	123	125	126	127	128
14	90th	119	120	121	122	124	125	126
	95th	123	124	125	126	128	129	130
15	90th	121	121	122	124	125	126	127
	95th	124	125	126	128	129	130	131
16	90th	122	122	123	125	126	127	128
	95th	125	126	127	128	130	131	132
17	90th	122	123	124	125	126	128	128
	95th	126	126	127	129	130	131	132

		Diastolic Blood Pressure by Percentile of Height, mm Hg†						
		5%	10%	25%	50%	75%	90%	95%
1	90th	53	53	53	54	55	56	56
	95th	57	57	57	58	59	60	60
2	90th	57	57	58	58	59	60	61
	95th	61	61	62	62	63	64	65
3	90th	61	61	61	62	63	63	64
	95th	65	65	65	66	67	67	68
4	90th	63	63	64	65	65	66	67
	95th	67	67	68	69	69	70	71
5	90th	65	66	66	67	68	68	69
	95th	69	70	70	71	72	72	73
6	90th	67	67	68	69	69	70	71
	95th	71	71	72	73	73	74	75

(continued)

BLOOD PRESSURE IN CHILDREN
(*Continued*)

Girls Age, y	Blood Pressure Percentile*	Diastolic Blood Pressure by Percentile of Height, mm Hg†						
		5%	10%	25%	50%	75%	90%	95%
7	90th	69	69	69	70	71	72	72
	95th	73	73	73	74	75	76	76
8	90th	70	70	71	71	72	73	74
	95th	74	74	75	75	76	77	78
9	90th	71	72	72	73	74	74	75
	95th	75	76	76	77	78	78	79
10	90th	73	73	73	74	75	76	76
	95th	77	77	77	78	79	80	80
11	90th	74	74	75	75	76	77	77
	95th	78	78	79	79	80	81	81
12	90th	75	75	76	76	77	78	78
	95th	79	79	80	80	81	82	82
13	90th	76	76	77	78	78	79	80
	95th	80	80	81	82	82	83	84
14	90th	77	77	78	79	79	80	81
	95th	81	81	82	83	83	84	85
15	90th	78	78	79	79	80	81	82
	95th	82	82	83	83	84	85	86
16	90th	79	79	79	80	81	82	82
	95th	83	83	83	84	85	86	86
17	90th	79	79	79	80	81	82	82
	95th	83	83	83	84	85	86	86

*Blood pressure percentile was determined by a single measurement.

†Height percentile was determined by standard growth curves.

Reproduced with permission from Update on the 1987 Task Force Report on High Blood Pressure in Children and Adolescents: A Working Group Report from the National High Blood Pressure Education Program. Pediatrics 98:649, 1996.

THE APICAL IMPULSE

	Normal	Hyperkinetic	Pressure Overload	Volume Overload
Location	5th or 4th left inter-space, inside midcla-vicular line	Normal	Normal	Displaced to the left and possibly downward
Diameter	Little more than 2 cm (1 cm in children); ≤3 cm when pa-tient lies on left side	Normal	Increased	Increased
Amplitude	Small, gently tapping	Increased	Increased	Increased
Duration	Less than $\frac{2}{3}$ of systole, stops before S_2	Normal	Prolonged, perhaps up to S_2	Often slightly prolonged
Examples of Causes		Anxiety, hyperthy-roidism, severe anemia	Hyper-tension, aortic stenosis	Aortic or mitral regurg-itation

HEART SOUNDS

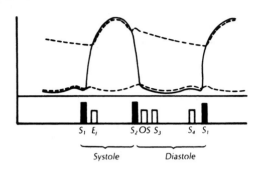

Finding	Possible Causes
S₁ Accentuated	Tachycardia, states of high cardiac output
	Mitral stenosis
S₁ Diminished	First-degree heart block
	Reduced left ventricular contractility
	Immobile mitral valve, as in mitral regurgitation
Ejection sound, aortic	Dilated aorta, aortic valve disease
Ejection sound, pulmonic	Dilated pulmonary artery, pulmonary hypertension, pulmonic stenosis
Systolic clicks(s)	Mitral valve prolapse
S₂ Accentuated in right 2nd interspace	Systemic hypertension, dilated aortic root
S₂ Diminished or absent in right 2nd interspace	Immobile aortic valve, as in calcific aortic stenosis
P₂ accentuated	Pulmonary hypertension, dilated pulmonary artery, atrial septal defect

(*continued*)

HEART SOUNDS

Finding	Possible Causes
P_2 diminished or absent	Aging, pulmonic stenosis
Opening snap	Mitral stenosis
S_3	Physiologic (usually in children and young adults)
	Pathologic myocardial failure, volume overload of a ventricle, as in mitral regurgitation
S_4	Excellent physical conditioning (trained athletes)
	Resistance to ventricular filling because of decreased compliance, as in hypertensive heart disease or coronary artery disease

AN APPARENTLY SPLIT FIRST HEART SOUND

	Split S$_1$	Aortic Ejection Sound	Early Systolic Click	Left-Sided S$_4$
Best heard at	Lower left sternal border	Right 2nd interspace, apex, or both	At or medial to apex or at left sternal border	Apex
Pitch	High	High	High	Low
Quality	Both components similar	Clicking	Clicking	Dull
Louder with	Diaphragm	Diaphragm	Diaphragm	Bell
Palpable split	Absent	Absent	Absent	May be present
Aids	None	None	Click delayed by squatting	Partial left lateral decubitus position

SPLITTING OF THE SECOND HEART SOUND

Physiologic Splitting increased in inspiration, usually disappears in expiration, especially if patient sits. A_2 precedes P_2.

Wide Splitting persistent through cardiac cycle and increases on inspiration. May be due to delayed P_2 (as in right bundle branch block, pulmonic stenosis) or early A_2 (as in mitral regurgitation).

Fixed Wide splitting that does not vary with respiration. Occurs in atrial septal defect, right ventricular failure.

Paradoxical Splitting that appears on expiration and disappears on inspiration. A_2 is abnormally delayed and follows P_2. Occurs in left bundle branch block.

HEART MURMURS AND SIMILAR SOUNDS

Likely Causes

Midsystolic

Innocent murmurs (no cardiovascular abnormality)

Physiologic murmurs (from increased flow across a semilunar valve, as in pregnancy, fever, anemia)

Aortic stenosis

Murmurs that mimic aortic stenosis (aortic sclerosis, bicuspid aortic valve, dilated aorta, and pathologically increased systolic flow across the aortic valve)

Hypertrophic cardiomyopathy

Pulmonic stenosis

Pansystolic

Mitral regurgitation

Tricuspid regurgitation

Ventricular septal defect

Late systolic

Mitral valve prolapse

Early diastolic

Aortic regurgitation

Middiastolic and presystolic

Mitral stenosis

(*continued*)

HEART MURMURS AND SIMILAR SOUNDS

Likely Causes

Continuous
murmurs and
murmurlike
sounds

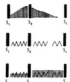

Patent ductus arteriosus

Pericardial friction rub (a scratchy
sound with 1–3 components)

Venous hum

CYANOSIS AND CONGENITAL HEART DISEASE

No Cyanosis	Early Cyanosis	Late Cyanosis
Small septal defects		Large septal defects
Mild pure pulmonic stenosis	Severe pulmonic stenosis with intact ventricular system	Mild pure pulmonic stenosis
Coarctation of the aorta	Severe tetralogy of Fallot	Less severe tetralogy of Fallot
Patent ductus arteriosus	Tricuspid atresia	Eisenmenger's complex
Anomalous origin of left coronary artery	Two- and three-chambered hearts	
Subendocardial fibroelastosis	Transposition of the great vessels	
Glycogen storage disease		

TENDER ABDOMENS

Visceral Tenderness	**Peritoneal Tenderness**

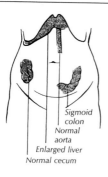

Sigmoid
colon
Normal
aorta
Enlarged liver
Normal cecum

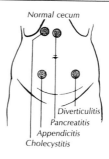

Normal cecum

Diverticulitis
Pancreatitis
Appendicitis
Cholecystitis

Tenderness From Disease in the Chest and Pelvis

Acute Pleurisy	*Acute Salpingitis*

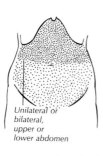

Unilateral or
bilateral,
upper or
lower abdomen

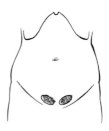

SEX MATURITY RATINGS IN GIRLS: BREASTS

Stage 1

Preadolescent—elevation of nipple only

Stage 2   **Stage 3**

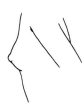   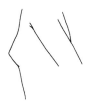

Breast bud stage. Elevation of   Further enlargement
breast and nipple as a small   and elevation of
mound; enlargement of   breast and areola,
areolar diameter   with no separation of
                                      the contours

Stage 4   **Stage 5**

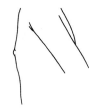   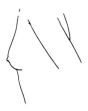

Projection of areola and   Mature stage;
nipple to form a secondary   projection of nipple
mound above the level of   only. Areola has
the breast   receded to general
                                      contour of the breast
                                      (although in some
                                      normal individuals
                                      areola continues to
                                      form a secondary
                                      mound).

(Illustrations through the courtesy of W. A. Daniel, Jr.)

SEX MATURITY RATINGS IN GIRLS: PUBIC HAIR

Stage 1

Preadolescent—no pubic hair except for the fine body hair (vellus hair) similar to that on the abdomen

Stage 2

Sparse growth of long, slightly pigmented, downy hair, straight or only slightly curled, chiefly along the labia

Stage 3

Darker, coarser, curlier hair, spreading sparsely over the pubic symphysis

Stage 4

Coarse and curly hair as in adults; area covered greater than in stage 3 but not as great as in the adult and not yet including the thighs

Stage 5

Hair adult in quantity and quality, spread on the medial surfaces of the thighs but not up over the abdomen

(Illustrations through the courtesy of W.A. Daniel, Jr.)

SEX MATURITY

In assigning SMRs in boys, observe each of the three characteristics separately. Record two separate ratings: pubic hair and genital. If the penis and testes differ in their stages, average the two into a single figure for the genital rating

Pubic Hair

Stage 1

Preadolescent—no pubic hair except for the fine body hair (vellus hair) similar to that on the abdomen

Stage 2

Sparse growth of long, slightly pigmented, downy hair, straight or only slightly curled, chiefly at the base of the penis

Stage 3

Darker, coarser, curlier hair spreading sparsely over the pubic symphysis

Stage 4

Coarse and curly hair, as in the adult; area covered greater than in stage 3 but not as great as in the adult and not yet including the thighs

Stage 5

Hair adult quantity and quality, spread to the medial surfaces of the thighs but not up over the abdomen

(Illustrations through the courtesy of W.A. Daniel, Jr.)

RATINGS IN BOYS

Genitalia

Penis	Testes and Scrotum
Preadolescent—same size and proportions as in childhood	Preadolescent—same size and proportions as in childhood
Slight to no enlargement	Testes larger; scrotum larger, somewhat reddened, and altered in texture
Larger, especially in length	Further enlarged
Further enlarged in length and breadth, with development of the glans	Further enlarged; scrotal skin darkened
Adult in size and shape	Adult in size and shape

ABNORMALITIES OF THE PENIS

Hypospadias	Congenital displacement of the urethral meatus to the inferior surface of the penis
Phimosis	A tight prepuce that cannot be retracted
Paraphimosis	A tight prepuce that, once retracted, cannot be replaced over the glans
Balanitis	Inflammation of the glans
Balanoposthitis	Inflammation of the glans and prepuce
Chancre	A usually nontender, firm erosion or ulcer, typically on the glans; due to primary syphilis
Genital herpes	A cluster of small vesicles, typically on the glans, that evolve into painful small ulcers on red bases
Venereal warts	Warty growths on the glans, shaft, or base of the penis; due to human papillomavirus
Cancer of the penis	An indurated and usually nontender nodule or ulcer of the glans or inner surface of the prepuce. Seen mainly in uncircumcised men

ABNORMALITIES IN THE SCROTUM

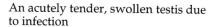

Scrotal hernia

Protrusion of abdominal contents through the external inguinal ring into the scrotum. The clinician's fingers cannot get above the mass.

Hydrocele

A fluid-filled sac in the tunica vaginalis. The clinician's fingers can get above the scrotal mass.

Acute orchitis

An acutely tender, swollen testis due to infection

Acute epididymitis

A tender, swollen epididymis, usually associated with infection of the urinary tract or prostate

Tuberculous epididymitis

Chronic inflammatory enlargement of the epididymis, often with thickening of the vas deferens

(continued)

ABNORMALITIES IN THE SCROTUM
(*Continued*)

Varicocele

Varicose veins of the spermatic cord, traditionally described as feeling like a "bag of worms."

Tumor of the testis

A usually painless, solid nodule or mass in the testis.

Cyst of the epididmyis

A small, painless, fluid-filled mass above the testis. A *spermatocele* is clinically like a cyst but contains sperm.

Torsion of the spermatic cord

An acutely tender, swollen testis due to twisting of the organ on the spermatic cord, with resulting circulatory impairment

Small testis

Small, firm testes suggest Klinefelter's syndrome; small, soft testis(es) suggest atrophy.

Cryptorchidism

An undescended testicle, not palpable in the scrotum. The scrotal sac is poorly developed on the involved side(s). Associated with increased risk of testicular carcinoma.

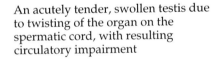

HERNIAS IN THE GROIN

Indirect inguinal

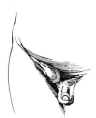

Most common hernia at all ages, both sexes. Originates above inguinal ligament and often passes into scrotum. May touch examiner's fingertip in inguinal canal

Direct inguinal

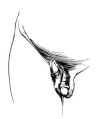

Less common than indirect hernia, usually occurs in men over age 40. Originates above inguinal ligament near external inguinal ring and rarely enters scrotum. May bulge anteriorly, touching side of examiner's finger

Femoral

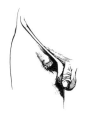

Least common hernia, more common in women than in men. Originates below inguinal ligament, more lateral than inguinal hernia. Never enters scrotum

ABNORMALITIES ON RECTAL EXAMINATION

 Cancer of the rectum. A firm to hard nodule or a rolled, irregular edge of an ulcerated cancer

 Polyp of the rectum. A soft mass that may or may not be on a stalk. May not be palpable

 Benign prostatic hyperplasia. An enlarged, nontender, smooth, firm but slightly elastic prostate gland. Benign prostatic hyperplasia can cause symptoms without palpable enlargement.

 Acute prostatitis. A prostate that is very tender, swollen, and firm because of acute infection

 Cancer of the prostate. A hard area in the prostate that may or may not feel nodular

ABNORMALITIES OF THE VULVA AND URETHRAL MEATUS

Ulcers of the vulva

SYPHILITIC CHANCRE	Usually firm and painless, often but not necessarily single
GENITAL HERPES	Painful, shallow, on red bases; usually several or multiple
ULCERATED CARCINOMA OF THE VULVA	Most common in elderly women but not limited exclusively to them

Raised lesions on the vulva

EPIDERMOID CYST. VENEREAL WARTS (CONDYLOMATA ACUMINATA)	Small, firm, round, smooth Irregular in surface (warty), often multiple
SECONDARY SYPHILIS (CONDYLOMATA LATA)	Slightly raised, flattened papules, round or oval, covered by a gray exudate
CARCINOMA OF THE VULVA	Raised, red, variable in appearance, may be ulcerated
BARTHOLIN'S GLAND INFECTION	A swelling in the posterior labium; tender and red when acute, cystic when chronic

Red swellings of the urethral meatus

URETHRAL CARUNCLE	A small swelling on the posterior aspect of the urethral meatus
PROLAPSED URETHRAL MUCOSA	A ring of swollen red mucosa surrounding the urethral meatus

VAGINITIS

	Discharge	Other Symptoms
Trichomonas vaginitis	Yellowish green, often profuse, may be malodorous	Itching, vaginal soreness, dyspareunia
Candida vaginitis	White, curdy, often thick, not malodorous	Itching, vaginal soreness, external dysuria, dyspareunia
Bacterial vaginosis	Gray or white, thin homogeneous, scant, malodorous	Fishy genital odor
Atrophic vaginitis	Variable in color, consistency, and amount; may be blood tinged; rarely profuse	Itching, dysuria, dyspareunia

VAGINITIS

Vulva	Vagina	Laboratory Assessment
May be red	May be normal or red, with red spots, petechiae	Saline wet mount for trichomonads
Often red and swollen	Often red with white patches of discharge	KOH preparation for branching hyphae
Usually normal	Usually normal	Saline wet mount for "clue cells," "whiff test" with KOH for fishy odor
Atrophic	Atrophic, dry, pale; may be red, petechial, ecchymotic; possible erosions or adhesions	

RELAXATIONS OF THE PELVIC FLOOR

When the pelvic floor is weakened, various structures may become displaced. These displacements are seen best when the patient strains down.

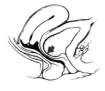

A cystocele is a bulge of the anterior wall of the upper part of the vagina, together with the urinary bladder above it.

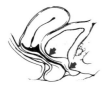

A cystourethrocele involves both the bladder and the urethra as they bulge into the anterior vaginal wall throughout most of its extent.

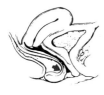

A rectocele is a bulge of the posterior vaginal wall, together with a portion of the rectum.

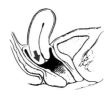

A prolapsed uterus has descended down the vaginal canal. There are three degrees of severity: first, still within the vagina (as illustrated); second, with the cervix at the introitus; and third, with the cervix outside the introitus.

COMMON VARIATIONS IN THE CERVIX

The os may be round, oval, or slitlike.

Lacerations from vaginal deliveries may be unilateral transverse, bilateral transverse, or stellate.

The epithelium of a normal cervix may be all squamous or both squamous and columnar. Retention (nabothian) cysts may be present.

Squamous   *Squamous*   *Cyst*
              Columnar

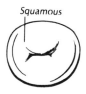 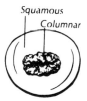 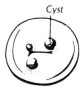

ABNORMALITIES OF THE CERVIX

Carcinoma of the cervix. An irregular, hard mass suggests cancer. Early lesions cannot be detected by physical examination alone.

Endocervical polyp. A bright red, smooth mass that protudes from the os suggests a polyp. It bleeds easily.

Mucopurulent cervicitis. A yellowish exudate emerging from the cervical os suggests this diagnosis. Causes include *Chlamydia* and gonococcal infections.

Columnar
epithelium *Vaginal
adenosis*
Collar

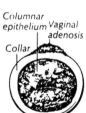

Fetal exposure to diethylstilbestrol. Several changes may be seen: a color of tissue around the cervix, columnar epithelium that covers the cervix or extends to the vaginal wall (then termed *vaginal adenosis*), and, rarely, carcinoma of the vagina.

POSITIONS OF THE UTERUS AND UTERINE MYOMAS

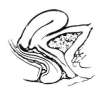

An anteverted uterus lies in a forward position at roughly a right angle to the vagina. This is the most common position. *Anteflexion*—a forward flexion of the uterine body in relation to the cervix—often coexists.

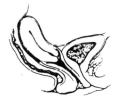

A retroverted uterus is tilted posteriorly with its cervix facing anteriorly.

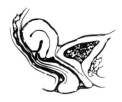

A retroflexed uterus has a posterior tilt that involves the uterine body but not the cervix. A uterus that is retroflexed or retroverted may be felt only through the rectal wall; some cannot be felt at all.

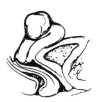

A myoma of the uterus is a very common, benign tumor that feels firm and often irregular. There may be more than one. A myoma on the posterior surface of the uterus may be mistaken for a retrodisplaced uterus; one on the anterior surface may be mistaken for an anteverted uterus.

THE DIAGNOSIS OF PREGNANCY

Suggestive symptoms in first trimester

No menstrual periods

Nausea with or without vomiting

Breast tenderness

Urinary frequency

Fatigue

Physical signs—in weeks from the last menstrual period

6 TO 8 WEEKS

Softening of the uterine isthmus—the first clinical manifestation of pregnancy (*Hegar's sign*)

Rounding of the body of the uterus into a globular shape

Softening of the cervix so that it feels like lips, not like the nose

Purplish color of the vaginal and cervical mucosa

12 WEEKS

Fetal heart audible with Doptone

18 WEEKS

Fetal heart audible with fetoscope

24 WEEKS

Fetal movements usually palpable by examiner

12 TO 36 WEEKS

A rise in the fundal height:

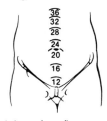

To calculate *expected date of confinement* (EDC): Add 7 days to the first day of last menstrual period, subtract 3 months, and add 1 year.

CHRONIC VASCULAR INSUFFICIENCY

	Arterial	Deep Venous
Pain	Intermittent claudication, possibly pain at rest	Aching on dependency
Pulses	Decreased or absent	Normal, but may be obscured by edema
Color	Pallor on elevation, rubor on dependency	Normal, or cyanotic on dependency. Pigmentation around the ankle
Temperature	Cool	Normal
Edema	Absent or mild	Present, often marked
Skin changes	Thin, shiny, atrophic; decreased hair; ridged, thickened nails	Brown pigment near the ankle, stasis dermatitis, and possible thickening of the skin with narrowing of the leg
Ulcers, if any	Toes, points of trauma	At the sides of the ankle, especially medially
Gangrene	May be present	Absent

PERIPHERAL CAUSES OF EDEMA

	Ortho-static Edema	Lymph-edema	Lip-edema	Deep Venous Insuffi-ciency
Edema	Soft, pitting	Soft early, becomes hard and non-pitting	Minimal, if any	Soft, pitting; may become hard and non-pitting
Skin thickening	Absent	Marked	Absent	Occasional
Ulceration	Absent	Rare	Absent	Common
Pigmentation	Absent	Absent	Absent	Common
Foot swelling	Yes	Yes	No	Yes
Bilaterality	Always	Often	Always	Occasional

ABNORMALITIES OF THE HANDS

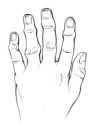

Osteoarthritis. Hard, dorsolateral nodules on the distal interphalangeal joints (*Heberden's nodes*) and, less commonly, similar nodules on the proximal interphalangeal joints (*Bouchard's nodes*)

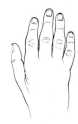

Acute rheumatoid arthritis. Tenderness, pain, stiffness, and swelling, affecting mainly the proximal interphalangeal and metacarpophalangeal joints

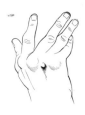

Chronic rheumatoid arthritis. Chronic swelling and thickening of the proximal interphalangeal and metacarpophalangeal joints; ulnar deviation of the fingers; muscular atrophy; rheumatoid nodules

Boutonnière (A) and *swan neck* (B) deformities may also be seen

(*continued*)

ABNORMALITIES OF THE HANDS
(Continued)

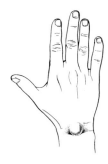

Ganglion. A cystic, round, usually nontender swelling along a tendon sheath or joint capsule. The wrist is a common site, but a ganglion may occur elsewhere.

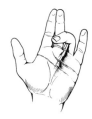

Dupuytren's contracture. A thickening of the palmar fascia, first felt as a nodule near the distal palmar crease. A fibrotic cord then develops, and a flexion contraction involving the finger may ensue.

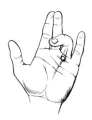

Trigger finger. A painless nodule in a flexor tendon of the palm, near the head of the metacarpal. Too big to slide easily into the tendon sheath on extension, it necessitates extra effort or force. A snap is felt and heard when it pops through.

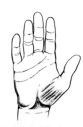

Thenar atrophy. Wasting of the muscles of the thenar eminence. It suggests a disorder of the median nerve.

SWOLLEN OR TENDER ELBOWS

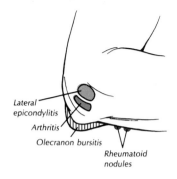

Epicondylitis	A painful, tender lateral epicondyle suggests *lateral epicondylitis* (tennis elbow). Extension of the wrist against resistance increases the pain.
	A painful, tender medial epicondyle (not illustrated) suggests *medial epicondylitis* (pitcher's, golfer's, or Little League elbow). Wrist flexion against resistance increases the pain.
Arthritis	Tenderness and swelling in the groove between the olecranon process and the lateral epicondyle suggest arthritis of the elbow joint.
Olecranon bursitis	Swelling superficial to the olecranon bursa suggests olecranon bursitis. It may be acute or chronic.
Rheumatoid nodules	Rheumatoid nodules are subcutaneous, firm, and nontender. They occur along the extensor surface of the ulna and may be attached to the underlying periosteum. They are associated with rheumatoid arthritis or acute rheumatic fever.

PAINFUL TENDER SHOULDERS

Acromioclavicular arthritis

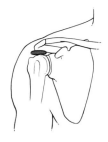

Tenderness over the acromioclavicular joint, especially with adduction of the arm across the chest, suggests acromioclavicular arthritis. Pain often increases with shrugging the shoulders. Usually results from direct injury to the shoulder girdle.

Subacromial and subdeltoid bursitis

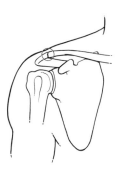

Pain over anterior superior aspect of shoulder, particularly when raising the arm overhead, suggests subacromial bursitis. Tenderness common anterolateral to the acromion, in hollow recess formed by the acromiohumeral sulcus. Often seen in overuse syndromes from repetitive motion as in pitching, swimming, or serving a tennis ball. Arises from impingement of the acromion, acromioclavicular ligament, and coracoid process against the underlying bursa, resulting in inflammation.

(continued)

PAINFUL TENDER SHOULDERS

Rotator cuff tendinitis

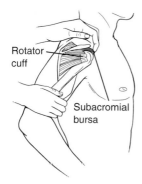

Tenderness over the rotator cuff, when elbow passively lifted posteriorly or with "drop arm" maneuver suggests rotator cuff tendinitis. Commonly occurs after age 50, begins with localized supraspinatus tendinitis, extends to other rotator cuff tendon insertions, and subacromial bursa. Can eventually involve the joint capsule, leading to a *frozen shoulder* from adhesive capsulitis. Arises from impingement of rotator cuff against undersurface of the acromion and coracoacromial ligament; may lead to inflammation and degenerative process of the rotator cuff tendons.

Bicipital tendinitis

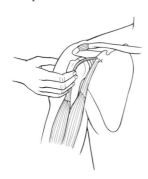

Tenderness over the long head of the biceps when rolled in the bicipital groove or when flexed arm is supinated against resistance suggests *bicipital tendinitis.*

PAINFUL TENDER KNEES

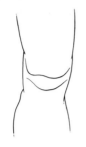

Arthritis.   *Degenerative arthritis* usually occurs after age 50; associated with obesity. Often with medial joint line tenderness, palpable osteophytes, bowleg appearance, mild effusion. Systemic involvement, swelling, and subcutaneous nodules in *rheumatoid arthritis*.

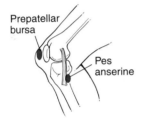

Prepatellar bursa

Pes anserine

Bursitis. Inflammation and thickening of bursa seen in repetitive motion and overuse syndromes. Can involve *prepatellar bursa* ("housemaid's knee"), *pes anserine* bursa medially (runners, osteoarthritis) *iliotibial band* laterally (over lateral femoral condyle), especially in runners.

(continued)

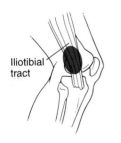

Iliotibial tract

PAINFUL TENDER KNEES

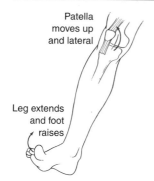

Patella moves up and lateral

Leg extends and foot raises

Patellofemoral instability. During flexion and extension of knee, due to subluxation and/or malalignment. Patella tracks laterally instead of centrally in the trochlear groove of distal femoral condyle. Inspect or palpate for lateral motion with leg extension. May lead to chondromalacia or osteoarthritis.

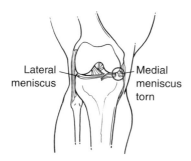

Lateral meniscus

Medial meniscus torn

Meniscal tear. Commonly arises from twisting injury of knee; in older patients may be degenerative. Patients report clicking, popping, or locking sensation. Check for tenderness along joint line over medial or lateral meniscus and for effusion. May be accompanied by associated tears of medial collateral or anterior cruciate ligaments.

(*continued*)

PAINFUL TENDER KNEES (Continued)

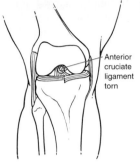

Anterior cruciate tear or sprain. Also seen in twisting injuries of the knee. Patients report popping sensation, immediate swelling, pain with flexion and extension, difficulty walking, and eventually the sensation of the knee "giving way." Check for anterior drawer sign, swelling from hemarthrosis, and for associated injuries to medial meniscus or medial collateral ligament. Consider evaluation by orthopedic surgery.

Anterior cruciate ligament torn

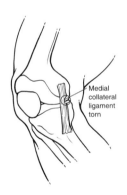

Collateral ligament sprain or tear. Often arises from force applied to medial or lateral surface of knee (valgus or varus stress respectively), producing localized swelling, pain, and stiffness. Patients usually able to walk but may develop an effusion later. Physical findings include tenderness over the affected ligament and ligamentous laxity during valgus or varus stress.

Medial collateral ligament torn

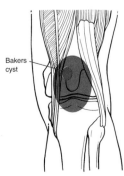

Baker's cyst. Cystic swelling palpable on the medial surface of the popliteal fossa, prompting complaints of aching or fullness behind the knee. Inspect and palpate for cystic swelling adjacent to the medial hamstring tendons. Presence of an effusion suggests involvement of the posterior horn of the medial meniscus. In rheumatoid arthritis cyst may expand into calf or even the ankle.

Bakers cyst

ABNORMALITIES OF THE FEET

Acute gouty arthritis. A hot, red, painful, and tender swelling often involving the first metatarsophalangeal joint.

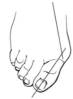

Hallux valgus. A lateral deviation of the great toe in relation to the first metatarsal, which itself may be deviated medially. A bursa may form between the metatarsal head and the skin and become inflamed (a bunion).

Hammer toe. Hyperextension at the metatarsophalangeal joint with flexion at the proximal interphalangeal joint.

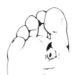

Plantar wart. A wart in the thick skin of the sole. It may be covered by a callus. Look for the small dark spots of a wart.

Neurotrophic ulcer. A painless, often deep ulcer typically surrounded by callus. It occurs at pressure points in diabetic and other patients whose pain sensation is decreased or absent.

Clubfoot (Talipes equinovarus). Characterized by forefoot adduction and by inversion and plantar flexion (equinus position) of the entire foot.

SPINAL CURVATURES

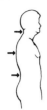

Normal. A cervical concavity, a thoracic convexity, and a lumbar concavity

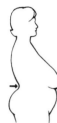

Lordosis. An accentuation of the normal lumbar concavity. It may accompany pregnancy, marked obesity, or kyphosis.

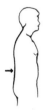

Flattening of the lumbar curve. Loss of the normal lumbar concavity. Causes include muscle spasm and ankylosing spondylitis.

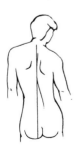

List. A lateral tilt of the spine. A plumb line dropped from T1 falls lateral to the gluteal cleft. Muscle spasm associated with a herniated disc is a common cause.

(*continued*)

SPINAL CURVATURES

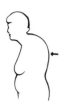

Kyphosis. An exaggerated, rounded thoracic convexity. It is common in aging, especially in women.

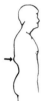

Gibbus. An angular, localized convexity due to one or more collapsed vertebrae. Causes include metastatic cancer and tuberculosis of the spine.

Scoliosis. A lateral curvature of the spine. It is described by the location and direction of its chief convexity, here a thoracic scoliosis with convexity to the right. Compensating curves usually correct any list.

Forward flexion often makes scoliosis more evident.

FACIAL PARALYSIS

	Lesion of Peripheral Nervous System	Lesion of Central Nervous System
Side of face affected	Same side as the lesion	Side opposite the lesion
Lower face e.g., smiling, showing teeth	Weak or paralyzed	Weak or paralyzed
Upper face, e.g., raising eyebrows, wrinkling forehead, closing eyes	Weak or paralyzed	Normal or slightly weak
Common cause	Bell's palsy (injury to CN VII)	Cerebrovascular accident

GAIT AND POSTURE

Spastic hemiparesis. Arm held close to the side with joints flexed. Leg extended and foot plantar flexed. On walking, the toe scrapes or the leg is circumducted.

Scissors gait (bilateral spastic paresis). A stiff gait in which the thighs cross forward on each other with each step. Steps are short.

Steppage gait (peripheral nerve weakness). Because of foot drop, either dragging of the feet or lifting them high and slapping them down

Sensory ataxia. Unsteady, wide-based gait, partially corrected by watching the ground. Feet thrown forward and outward and brought down on heels and then toes. Romberg test positive

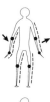

Cerebellar ataxia. Unsteady, wide-based gait, with special difficulty on turns. In Romberg test, unsteadiness with eyes open or closed. Other cerebellar signs are associated.

Parkinsonism. Stooped posture with flexed elbows and wrists. Slow, shuffling gait with short steps and stiff turns

MOTOR DISORDERS

	Peripheral Nervous System Disorder	Central Nervous System Disorder*
Involuntary movements	Often fasciculations	No fasciculations
Muscle bulk	Atrophy	Normal or mild atrophy (disuse)
Muscle tone	Decreased or absent	Increased, spastic
Muscle strength	Decreased or lost	Decreased or lost
Coordination	Unimpaired, though limited by weakness	Slowed and limited by weakness
Reflexes		
Deep tendon	Decreased or absent	Increased
Plantar	Flexor or absent	Extensor
Abdominals	Absent	Absent

Upper motor neuron

Parkinsonism (Basal Ganglia Disorder)	Cerebellar Disorder
Resting tremors	Intention tremors
Normal	Normal
Increased, rigid	Decreased
Normal or slightly decreased	Normal or slightly decreased
Good, though slowed and often tremulous	Impaired, ataxic
Normal or decreased	Normal or decreased
Flexor	Flexor
Normal	Normal

INVOLUNTARY MOVEMENTS

Tremors. Rhythmic oscillations that may be most evident (1) on movement (intention), (2) at rest, or (3) when maintaining a posture

INTENTION TREMORS

RESTING TREMORS

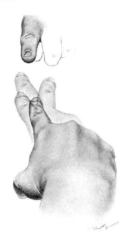

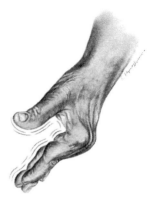

POSTURAL TREMORS

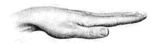

Fasciculations. Fine, rapid flickering of muscle bundles

Chorea. Brief, rapid, irregular, jerky; face, head, arms, or hands

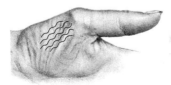

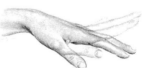

(continued)

INVOLUNTARY MOVEMENTS

Athetosis. Slow, twisting, writhing; face, distal limbs

Dystonia. Grotesque, twisted postures, often in trunk or, as shown, in neck (*spasmodic torticollis*)

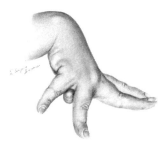

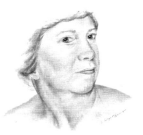

Tics. Brief, irregular, repetitive, coordinated movements, e.g., winking, shrugging

Oral–facial dyskinesias. Rhythmic, repetitive, bizarre movements of face, mouth

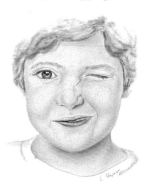

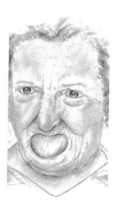

DERMATOMES

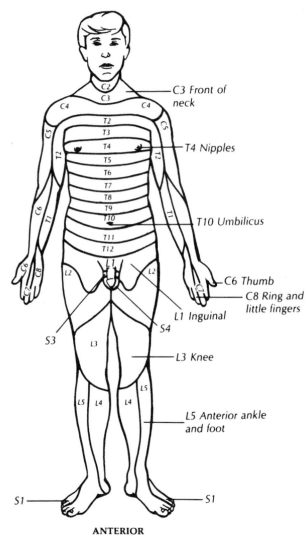

C3 Front of neck

T4 Nipples

T10 Umbilicus

C6 Thumb

C8 Ring and little fingers

L1 Inguinal

L3 Knee

L5 Anterior ankle and foot

ANTERIOR

(continued)

DERMATOMES

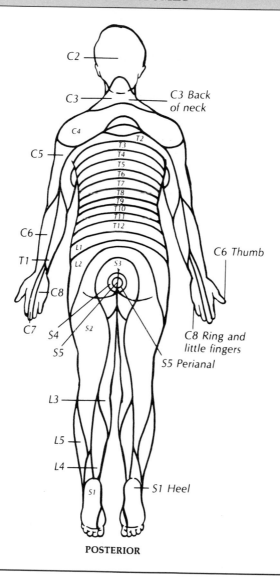

POSTERIOR

ABNORMAL POSTURES IN COMA

Decorticate rigidity

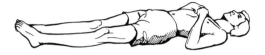

Occurs in lesions of corticospinal tracts in or near the cerebral hemispheres. When unilateral, this is the posture of chronic spastic hemiplegia.

Decerebrate rigidity

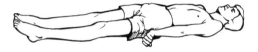

Occurs in severe metabolic coma or in structural coma involving the diencephalon, midbrain, or pons

Flaccid hemiplegia

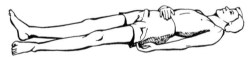

Occurs early in the course of unilateral lesions of the corticospinal tract

METABOLIC AND STRUCTURAL COMA

	Metabolic	Structural
Respiratory Pattern	If regular, normal or hyperventilation. If irregular, Cheyne–Stokes	Irregular, especially Cheyne–Stokes or ataxic breathing
Pupils	Equal, reactive to light. (If pinpoint, use magnifier.) May be fixed, dilated from anticholinergics, hypothermia	Unequal or unreactive to light. Midposition and fixed in midbrain compression. Dilated and fixed in compression of cranial nerve III by herniation
Level of consciousness	Changes after pupils change	Changes before pupils change
Causes Include:	Uremia, liver failure Alcohol, drugs	Epidural, subdural, intracerebral hemorrhage
	Hypothyroidism	Cerebral infarct or embolus
	Anoxia, ischemia	Tumor, abscess
	Meningitis, encephalitis	Lesion in brainstem or cerebellum
	Hyper- or hypothermia	
	Hyper- or hypoglycemia	

ATTRIBUTES OF CLINICAL DATA

Validity—the closeness with which a measurement reflects the true value of an object

Reliability—the reproducibility of a measurement

Sensitivity, specificity, and *predictive values* are illustrated in a 2 × 2 table, as shown below in an example of 200 people, half of whom have the disease in question. A prevalence of 50% is much higher than is usually found in a clinical situation. Because the positive predictive value increases with prevalence, its calculated value here is accordingly and unrealistically high.

		Disease		
		Present	**Absent**	
	+	**95** true positive observations *a*	*b* **10** false positive observations	**105** total positive observations
Observation				
	−	**5** false negative observations *c*	*d* **90** true negative observations	**95** total negative observations
		100 total persons with the disease	**100** total persons without the disease	**200** total persons

$$\text{Sensitivity} = \frac{a}{a+c} = \frac{95}{95+5} \times 100 = 95\%$$

$$\text{Specificity} = \frac{d}{b+d} = \frac{90}{90+10} \times 100 = 90\%$$

$$\text{Positive predictive value} = \frac{a}{a+b} = \frac{95}{95+10} \times 100 = 90.5\%$$

$$\text{Negative predictive value} = \frac{d}{c+d} = \frac{90}{90+5} \times 100 = 94.7\%$$

CLINICAL THINKING AND THE PATIENT'S RECORD

Three parts of the patient's record are outlined in this chapter: (1) a comprehensive evaluation of an adult, from the history to the plan for the patient, (2) a problem list, and (3) a progress note. Clinical thinking is reviewed in the assessment portion of the comprehensive evaluation. Details of the history (see Chap. 1) are not repeated here. Major items in the physical examination are listed and should be expanded as indicated for a particular patient.

HISTORY

IDENTIFYING DATA, including name, address, age, place of birth, marital status, race, occupation, and religion

REFERRAL SOURCE, if any

SOURCE OF HISTORY

RELIABILITY, if relevant

CHIEF COMPLAINT(S)

PRESENT ILLNESS, including

A chronologic account of the symptoms and their attributes
The meaning of the illness to the patient and his or her responses to it
Current medications, including home remedies, prescription and nonprescription drugs, vitamin/mineral supplements
Allergies

PAST HISTORY

General health, as the patient perceives it
Childhood illnesses
Adult illnesses, including medical, surgical, obstetric,
    gynecologic, and psychiatric illnesses
Injuries
Transfusions

CURRENT HEALTH STATUS

Tobacco
Alcohol/drugs
Screening tests
Immunizations
Sleep
Exercise and diet, including daily intake, restrictions,
    supplements
Safety measures and environmental hazards

FAMILY HISTORY in diagrammatic or outline form. This should give the age and medical condition of at least the parents, siblings, spouse, and children, and the age at death, with its cause, of any who have died.

The symbols and structure of a family diagram are shown in the figure below:

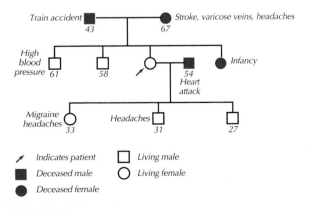

The family history should also include common familial or hereditary diseases and the presence of an illness similar to the patient's in any family member.

PSYCHOSOCIAL HISTORY

Education
Home situation, significant others, and daily life
Important past experiences, such as school, work,
    marriage(s)
Outlook on the present and the future
Relevant religious beliefs

REVIEW OF SYSTEMS

General, including weight, weakness, fatigue, and fever
Skin
Head
Eyes
Ears
Nose and sinuses
Mouth and throat
Neck
Breasts
Respiratory
Cardiac
Gastrointestinal
Urinary
Genital
Peripheral vascular
Musculoskeletal
Neurologic
Hematologic
Endocrine
Psychiatric

PHYSICAL EXAMINATION

General survey, described in a succinct paragraph
Vital signs. Pulse rate, respiratory rate, blood pressure, and
    possibly temperature
Height and weight, in gown if possible
Skin. Color, texture, lesions; hair and nails

Head. Hair, scalp, skull, face

Eyes. Vision, visual fields; conjunctiva, sclera; cornea, iris, lens; pupils (size, shape, reactions to light), extraocular movements; ophthalmoscopic examination

Ears. Auricles, canals, drums, auditory acuity, and, if indicated, Weber and Rinne tests

Nose. Mucosa, septum, sinus tenderness

Mouth. Lips, oral mucosa, gums, teeth, tongue, pharynx

Neck. Thyroid gland, trachea

Lymph nodes. Cervical, axillary, epitrochlear, inguinal

Thorax/lungs. Breathing (pattern, effort, sound), shape of chest, fremitus, percussion note, breath sounds, adventitious (added) sounds

Cardiovascular. Carotid pulses, jugular venous pressure, apical impulse, heart sounds, extra sounds, heart murmurs

Breasts. Size, symmetry, tenderness, masses

Abdomen. Shape, scars. Bowel sounds. Percussion note and pattern. Tenderness, including costovertebral angle tenderness; masses. Liver, spleen, kidneys, aorta

Genitalia

- Male. Penis, scrotum and contents, including testes; hernias
- Female. Vulva, vagina, cervix, uterus (size, shape, position), adnexa. Rectovaginal examination

Rectum. Anus, rectum, and (in men) prostate. Stool for occult blood.

Peripheral vascular. Skin color, peripheral pulses, edema, varicose veins

Musculoskeletal. Deformities, swollen or tender joints. Back (curvatures or tenderness). Range of motion

Neurologic

- Mental status: including orientation to person, place, time. Further detail as indicated, such as behavior, speech, and language, mood, thought and perception, memory and attention, higher cognitive functions.
- Cranial nerves (not already described)
- Motor system: body position, involuntary movements, muscle bulk, muscle tone, strength; cerebellar function, including coordination (rapid alternating movements, point-to-point movements), gait and stance (Romberg test, pronator drift)

- Sensory system: pain, light touch, position, vibration, discriminative senses
- Reflexes, including Babinski sign

ASSESSMENT

For each problem identified from the patient's history, physical examination, or laboratory studies, summarize the relevant data and outline the clinical thinking that led to your formulation. The steps in the thought processes involved in this assessment are outlined below.

- Identify and list the abnormal findings in the data base, including symptoms, physical findings, and laboratory data.
- Cluster these findings into logical groups.
- Localize the findings anatomically as precisely as the data allow.
- Interpret the findings in terms of probable process.
- Make one or more hypotheses about the nature of the patient's problems.
- Eliminate hypotheses that do not explain the key findings or that are incompatible with them.
- Weigh the probability of competing hypotheses according to: their match with the findings; their probability in this particular patient (of the given age, sex, habits, geographic location, and other variables)
- Consider carefully the possibility of potentially life-threatening or treatable conditions even if they are less common and thus less likely.
- Establish a working definition of the problem(s) at the highest level of certainty and explicitness that the data allow.
- Recall that various findings can be evaluated according to their validity, reliability, sensitivity, specificity, and predictive values. Definitions of these terms are given on p. 246.

PLAN

For each problem, develop a plan in three categories:

- Diagnostic
- Therapeutic
- Educational

PROBLEM LIST

This is a numbered list of problems that is usually placed in the front of the patient's chart. The name of a problem (but not its number) is modified if additional data change the assessment. In the following example, the clinician crossed out "Edema, left leg" after making the new, more precise diagnosis of deep venous thrombosis.

Date problem entered	No.	Active problems	Inactive problems
9-24-94	1.	~~Edema, left leg~~	
9-25-94	1.	Deep venous thrombosis, left iliofemoral vein	
9-25-94	2.	Acute chest pain and dyspnea	

PROGRESS NOTE

Include the date and perhaps the time. Give the number and name of the problem, followed by

- S. (Subjective) The patient's report
- O. (Objective) The clinician's observations
- A. (Assessment) The clinician's interpretation of what is going on
- P. (Plan) Further plans, diagnostic, therapeutic, or educational

INDEX